COMMITTEE TO REVIEW THE CDC CENTERS FOR RESEARCH AND DEMONSTRATION OF HEALTH PROMOTION AND DISEASE PREVENTION

LAWRENCE W. GREEN (Chair), Director, Institute for Health Promotion Research, and Professor of Health Care and Epidemiology, University of British Columbia, Vancouver, British Columbia, Canada

NOREEN M. CLARK, Dean and Marshall H. Becker Professor of Public Health, University of Michigan, Ann Arbor, Michigan

JOHN W. FARQUHAR,* Director, Stanford Center for Research in Disease Prevention, and Professor of Medicine, Health Research and Policy, Stanford University, Palo Alto, California

MARY DESVIGNES-KENDRICK, Director, Houston Department of Health and Human Services, Houston, Texas

IRA S. MOSCOVICE, Professor and Associate Director, Institute for Health Services Research, School of Public Health, University of Minnesota, Minneapolis, Minnesota

JAMES O. PROCHASKA, Director, Cancer Prevention Research Center, and Professor of Psychology, University of Rhode Island, Kingston, Rhode Island

RANDY H. SCHWARTZ, Director, Division of Community and Family Health, Maine Department of Human Services, Bureau of Health, Augusta, Maine

LEE SECHREST, Professor, Department of Psychology, University of Arizona, Tucson, Arizona

HAROLD C. SOX, JR.,* Chair, Department of Medicine, and Joseph M. Huber Professor of Medicine, Dartmouth Medical School, Lebanon, New Hampshire

KENNETH E. WARNER,* Richard D. Remington Collegiate Professor of Public Health, University of Michigan, Ann Arbor, Michigan

IOM Staff

Michael A. Stoto, Director, Division of Health Promotion and Disease Prevention

Linda A. Bailey, Study Director (until September 1996)

Donna Thompson, Administrative Assistant

---

*Member, Institute of Medicine.

Linking Research and Public Health Practice

A Review of CDC's Program of Centers for Research and Demonstration of Health Promotion and Disease Prevention

Michael A. Stoto, Lawrence W. Green,
and Linda A. Bailey, Editors

Committee to Review the CDC Centers for Research and
Demonstration of Health Promotion and Disease Prevention

Board on Health Promotion and Disease Prevention

INSTITUTE OF MEDICINE

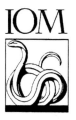

NATIONAL ACADEMY PRESS
Washington, D.C. 1997

NATIONAL ACADEMY PRESS • 2101 Constitution Avenue, N.W. • Washington, D.C. 20418

NOTICE: The project that is the subject of this report was approved by the Governing Board of the National Research Council, whose members are drawn from the councils of the National Academy of Sciences, the National Academy of Engineering, and the Institute of Medicine. The members of the committee responsible for the report were chosen for their special competences and with regard for appropriate balance.

This report has been reviewed by a group other than the authors according to procedures approved by a Report Review Committee consisting of members of the National Academy of Sciences, the National Academy of Engineering, and the Institute of Medicine.

The Institute of Medicine was chartered in 1970 by the National Academy of Sciences to enlist distinguished members of the appropriate professions in the examination of policy matters pertaining to the health of the public. In this, the Institute acts under the Academy's 1863 congressional charter responsibility to be an adviser to the federal government and its own initiative in identifying issues of medical care, research, and education. Dr. Kenneth I. Shine is president of the Institute of Medicine.

Funding for this project was provided by the Centers for Disease Control and Prevention, U.S. Department of Health and Human Services (contract no. 200-95-0964). The views presented in this report are those of the Committee to Review the CDC Centers for Research and Demonstration of Health Promotion and Disease Prevention and are not necessarily those of the funding organization.

International Standard Book No. 0-309-05680-2.

First Printing, January 1997

Second Printing, May 1997

Additional copies of this report are available for sale from the National Academy Press, Box 285, 2101 Constitution Avenue, N.W., Washington DC 20055. Call (800) 624-6242 or (202) 334-3313 (in the Washington Metropolitan area), or visit the NAP's on-line bookstore at **http://www.nap.edu/bookstore.**

The serpent has been a symbol of long life, healing, and knowledge among almost all cultures and religions since the beginning of recorded history. The image adopted as a logotype by the

Preface

In 1986, Congress authorized the Centers for Disease Control and Prevention (CDC) to develop a program of university-based research centers to undertake research projects in health promotion and disease prevention and to demonstrate the use of new and innovative research in public health techniques to improve public health. A decade later, after the prevention research center program grew from 3 initial centers to 13, the director of the CDC Division of Adult and Community Health, which oversees the program, requested of the Institute of Medicine (IOM) an evaluation of the overall program. To execute this study, the IOM established the Committee to Review the CDC Centers for Research and Demonstration of Health Promotion and Disease Prevention, which has prepared this report.

The broad mission of the prevention research centers program—to contribute to a fuller understanding of how the health of communities, and the nation, can be improved—can be achieved only through the sustained cooperation of a diverse array of professionals and nonprofessionals who have roles in influencing the health of communities, who have competing goals and priorities, and who have little history of engaging in long-term, cooperative efforts. Consistent with this understanding, the committee took a broad view of how prevention research can influence the health of communities, considering not only the proximal risk factors for disease prevention, but also the more distal conditions for health promotion and improved equity in the distribution of risk factors.

On a practical level, the committee recognized the difficulty of conducting community-based prevention research. The committee examined how a prevention research center could foster collaboration among these different groups and overcome the barriers separating universities from their surrounding communities. It also considered the need for high-quality research that produces research findings relevant to other communities, states, and regions.

The committee brought together expertise in prevention research, behavioral sciences, preventive medicine, clinical medicine, community health, health promotion and education, rural health, health services research, research administration, evaluation sciences, epidemiology, and public health practice at the state and local levels. Committee members met three times between March and July 1996. CDC staff and some of those who advocated for the program while it was being considered by the Congress joined the committee for its first meeting.

In addition to its regular meetings, members of the committee and its staff conducted site visits to prevention research centers in New York, North Carolina, and New Mexico, and to the CDC offices in Atlanta responsible for the direction and funding of the program. The director of the prevention research center at the University of Washington met with the committee during its July meeting. Telephone interviews, following detailed review of documents and written responses, were conducted with senior staff of the remaining nine centers. Informal contacts were made with others, including public health officials in the states and localities in which the centers are located. The site visits, meetings, reports, and telephone interviews gave the committee the opportunity to discuss important issues with prevention research center researchers and their collaborators, such as the challenges of developing innovative research projects, conducting demonstration projects in underserved communities, improving public health practices, and disseminating research findings.

The committee is grateful for the input it received from many individuals at its meetings, during site visits, in writing, and in other ways. The prevention research center directors and co-directors and the CDC staff who responded to the committee's surveys and participated in site visits are listed in Appendix C. Bo Barrow, Don Benken, Roger Bulger, Michael Eriksen, Patricia Evans, Michael Gemmell, D.A. Henderson, Martha Katz, Lloyd Kolbe, James Marks, David McQueen, Gil Omenn, and Jean Smith participated in the committee's meetings or provided information for the committee. Patricia Riley, the CDC program director, was especially generous of her time and energy. The committee also thanks the IOM staff responsible for the project, including Linda Bailey, who was responsible for organizing the committee's meeting, site visits, and interviews, and for background research and writing; Donna Thompson, for project assistance; Marnie Muscoplat and Kimberly Tremel, who provided research support; and Michael Stoto, the director of the IOM Division of Health Promotion and Disease Prevention, in which this project was housed.

In this report the committee concludes that the CDC prevention research centers program has had substantial progress and its participants are to be commended for its contributions to health promotion and disease prevention. The report proposes a set of recommendations intended to strengthen the quality and management of the program as it begins its second decade of work. By strengthening the program, the prevention research centers can contribute even more to local, state, and national efforts to improve the health of Americans.

Lawrence W. Green, *Chair*

Contents

Linking Research and Public Health Practice

A Review of CDC's Program of Centers for Research and Demonstration of Health Promotion and Disease Prevention

Executive Summary

Health promotion and disease prevention are central priorities in the Centers for Disease Control and Prevention (CDC) vision, *Healthy People In A Healthy World Through Prevention* (CDC, n.d.). To advance research in these areas, Congress authorized and CDC established a program of university-based Centers for Research and Demonstration of Health Promotion and Disease Prevention. Congress authorized the program to "undertake research and demonstration projects in health promotion, disease prevention, and improved methods of appraising health hazards and risk factors, and shall serve as demonstration sites for the use of new and innovative research in public health technique to improve public health" (PL 98-551). The prevention research centers (PRC) program[1] began in 1986 with funding to three universities. With periodic competitive renewals and expansions of the program, there are now 13 PRCs.[2]

Multidisciplinary faculty at these PRCs, located at schools of public health and academic health centers, focus on a series of related projects on a public health theme defined in terms of special populations, risk factors, or specific health conditions. The PRCs are expected to form partnerships to develop

---

[1]Public Law 98-551 created Centers for Research and Demonstration of Health Promotion and Disease Prevention. Throughout this report, the committee refers to these university-based centers as prevention research centers, or PRCs. In referring to the administration of the program by CDC, the committee uses the terminology "the PRC program."

[2]A 14th PRC grant was awarded after the committee completed its final meeting.

1

innovative ways to prevent disease and promote health, focus on high-priority public health issues, and conduct research and demonstration activities that result in improved public health practice. The PRCs are intended to serve as bridges between science and practice, and from academia to state and local health departments, health care providers and provider organizations, and community organizations, as well as with CDC. Evaluation research is embedded in many of the PRC interventions, and the centers also train public health professionals in applied prevention research.

PL 98-551 authorized the Secretary of Health and Human Services to provide annual funding at the level of $1 million per center for a total of 3 centers in 1985, 8 centers in 1986, and 13 centers in 1987. The actual annual appropriations from Congress, however, have fallen short of these authorization levels. Since the program was established, Congress has expanded the core PRC program from a total budget of $1.5 million to a total budget of approximately $7 million in fiscal year 1995. In 1993, CDC began providing supplementary funds to the PRCs through a Special Interest Project (SIP) funding mechanism as a way to increase the levels of research activity within the PRCs. The PRCs received a total of $9.5 million through SIP funding in 1995.

CHARGE TO THE COMMITTEE

In 1995, CDC asked the Institute of Medicine (IOM) to review the PRC program to examine the extent to which the program is providing the public health community with workable strategies to address major public health problems in disease prevention and health promotion. IOM established a 10-member committee to evaluate the PRC program. CDC asked the committee to evaluate (1) the overall quality and appropriateness of the health promotion and disease prevention research and demonstration projects being carried out at the PRCs and (2) CDC's management and oversight of the PRC program. The committee has not assessed the quality of the health promotion and disease prevention research and demonstration projects of individual PRCs. No comprehensive evaluation of the individual PRCs has ever been done. Rather, the focus is on CDC's plans, actions, evaluation and support of the overall PRC program.

A VISION FOR THE PREVENTION CENTERS RESEARCH PROGRAM

The committee's review and discussions with some of those associated with the development of the PRC program indicate that there are at least three ways in which the PRC program can serve CDC's purposes. First, in fulfillment of its mission as the nation's prevention agency, CDC could use the PRC program to undertake the research and development that any successful, forward-looking science-based agency must have. An increasing number of researchers are recognizing the importance of community factors among the determinants of health and the consequent potential for community-based interventions, as well as the value of community involvement in the conduct of health research—that is, setting the research goal or question, developing community-appropriate methodology, interpreting results, and disseminating findings. Through the PRC program, CDC could lead the way in generating needed knowledge about this new, community-based approach to research.

Second, CDC could use the PRC program as a way to build capacity for public health practice outside its Atlanta headquarters. The university-based PRCs, which have collaborative relationships with state and local health departments, community organizations, and other entities, might serve as extensions of CDC's Atlanta-based activities in field settings that would otherwise be beyond the agency's reach.

Finally, CDC could use the PRC program as a way to work with disadvantaged communities—those with high proportions of poor and underserved individuals—on critical public health problems. By focusing its research efforts on issues relevant to particular disadvantaged communities associated with the PRCs, the program could develop new knowledge appropriate to similar communities nationwide.

As any complex program must, the PRC program needs to establish a vision for the future to allow it to succeed as it moves into its second decade. Many options are available. The vision should encourage PRCs and others who work in health promotion and disease prevention to expand their activities, evolving toward centers characterized by:

- focus on risk conditions and social determinants of health;
- an orientation toward the community;
- interdisciplinarity;
- a means for dissemination research in public health;
- an interactive process for establishing research priorities;
- a role in setting national research priorities.

THE RESEARCH AND DEMONSTRATION PROJECTS CONDUCTED BY THE PREVENTION RESEARCH CENTERS

The value of the PRC program is largely determined by the content and the quality of the research and demonstration projects conducted by the PRCs. The committee assessed the contribution of the PRCs' efforts in innovation, setting priorities, and dissemination and implementation activities.

Innovation

A research project could be judged innovative if it addressed an underserved or previously unreached population, or if it were to test previously tested methods on a different but important health problem. In these terms, the committee found that the research and demonstration projects conducted by the PRCs were indeed innovative.

The PRCs were less innovative in the area of research methodology and the development of new interventions. One way to enhance a PRC's ability to develop new interventions and research methods is to establish a methodology unit or otherwise identify a group of PRC personnel that is responsible for methodological development. Methodology units of this sort are also likely to increase the PRC's ability to raise research funding from sources other than CDC. Thus, the committee recommends that

 • **PRCs should include methodology units or assigned personnel in support of research methods development as a core activity.**

Setting Priorities in the PRCs

In its interviews, site visits, and record reviews, the committee found little evidence of explicit criteria for selecting research projects in the individual PRCs. Specific criteria can help any research center set a coherent direction, and they can also improve the quality of the individual research projects selected. Thus, the committee recommends that

 • **PRCs should clearly state their criteria for project selection and evaluation.**

The committee's review of the research portfolios of the individual PRCs suggests that the quality of research and demonstration projects that are being conducted is highly variable. Most of the PRCs do not have a well-defined process for evaluating the results of their research projects. The quality of research and demonstration projects may be enhanced by an internal quality control mechanism for reports, publications, research proposals, and other PRC products. Thus, the committee recommends that

• **PRCs should have an internal quality control mechanism such as a review panel for reports, publications, research proposals, and other PRC products.**

Peer-reviewed publications are an important means of reviewing the quality of projects as well as an important means of disseminating new knowledge in professional communities. The committee finds that, as a group, the PRCs produce too few peer-reviewed research publications relative to their resources and their maturity; PRCs should be encouraged to publish their findings in the peer-reviewed literature. Therefore, the committee recommends that

• **More of the findings of the PRCs should be published in the peer reviewed scientific literature.**

There are examples of projects that have had a clear impact on the community's health, as well as policies and practices in public health agencies, health service delivery systems, and other community organizations concerned about public health. The committee's impression, however, is that relatively few of the research efforts have produced an impact that reaches beyond the immediate community. To clarify the impact of the PRCs' research, the committee recommends that

• **PRCs should document the impact of their activities on public health research, practice, and policy, both locally and nationally.**

CDC has an opportunity to advance the science of community-based research through the PRC program. The committee's review of the individual PRCs, however, indicated that some are more oriented to this approach than others. Thus, the committee recommends that

• **The PRCs should adopt a community-based approach to their research and demonstration efforts.**

Dissemination and Implementation Activities

Research findings and products from the PRCs and CDC should be disseminated to all PRCs, their communities, and their regional populations; to the research and professional communities through scientific and professional literature; to the public health practice community; and to the general public. Thus, the committee recommends that

• **The PRC program, as a whole, should increase its focus on dissemination efforts.**

The impact of the PRC program can be enhanced through cooperative dissemination activities among the PRCs and between the network of PRCs and other health promotion organizations such as state and local health departments in the United States and elsewhere. Thus, the committee recommends that

• **PRCs should seek to be part of regional and national networks for prevention that include CDC, the public health practice community, and other relevant parties.**

In reviewing the activities of the PRCs, the committee found many instances of dissemination activities, but few projects focused on dissemination research. Since the university-based PRCs are attempting a variety of dissemination approaches to a wide array of public and professional audiences, and because academic institutions have some research capacity, they are in a unique position to carry out dissemination research. Thus, the committee recommends that

• **The PRCs should increase their dissemination *research* efforts.**

MANAGEMENT AND OVERSIGHT OF THE PREVENTION RESEARCH CENTERS PROGRAM

Vision and Goals

Through their research and demonstration activities, the PRCs can—and have—made significant contributions toward meeting some of the national goals and objectives of *Healthy People 2000* (USDHHS, 1991). CDC's strategic plan (CDC, 1994) makes mention of the PRC program, but it does not appear to feature the program as a resource or asset. To ensure that the PRC program remains relevant to critical current public health issues, the committee recommends that

• **CDC should ensure that the vision and goals of the PRC program are compatible, mutually supportive, and consistent with the agency's overall strategic plan and with *Healthy People 2000*. The PRC program's vision and goals should define, in a clear and comprehensive way, the contributions of the PRC program to national priorities.**

CDC defines prevention research in the application guidelines for the PRC program as research designed "to yield results *directly applicable* to interventions to prevent occurrence of disease and disability, or the progression of detectable but asymptomatic disease." This definition, however, should not be interpreted as limiting the scope of research to disease prevention priorities, and it should include health promotion. In order that the PRC program remain consistent with current theory and practice in health promotion and disease prevention, the committee recommends that

• **CDC should modify its definition of *prevention research* as articulated in the application guidelines for the PRC program to encompass the broader scope of health promotion research that is needed to address the underlying determinants of health (risk conditions) and to build the capacity of individuals and communities to "cultivate health," rather than to focus solely on those determinants with immediate application to disease prevention (risk factors).**

Thematic Focus

An academic center is more likely to build a cohesive program of research and to have a major impact on public health problems when the center develops a strong sense of its own identity. PRCs, however, are faced with a dynamic tension between criteria based on their themes and those defined by the SIP program and other funding opportunities. In order to clarify CDC's expectations regarding the PRC program's contributions, the committee recommends that

• **CDC should provide guidance to the PRCs about the role of the PRCs' themes in selecting core research and demonstration projects and SIPs.**

CDC's Role in Networking, Communication, and Dissemination

The PRC program can enhance prevention research and the public's health through improved communication and networking mechanisms. To achieve this goal, each PRC should be called upon periodically to report what it has learned that is new and warrants replication or adaptation and evaluation in other PRCs that serve different populations. In order to consolidate the information for public health policy being gained from the PRC program, the committee recommends that

• **CDC should provide more opportunities for the PRCs to meet collectively, share lessons learned, exchange information related to findings, activate their collective communication channels on behalf of worthy projects, and provide mutual support, especially from strong PRCs to fledgling centers.**

The added value of the PRC program is its focus on community-based research, and CDC should encourage the public health practice community and other agencies and sectors to take greater advantage of the resource represented by the PRCs in their region and elsewhere. Thus, to foster better connections between the PRCs and the communities they work with, the committee recommends that

• **CDC should develop strategies for improving community input into the PRCs.**

PRCs have not exchanged information in a systematic way, and opportunities for replication of investigations into dissemination and implementation have not been exploited. PRCs have not regularly and systematically reported their findings concerning dissemination and implementation to CDC, and CDC does not have a mechanism for assembling findings from the various PRCs in order to promote such activities. Thus, to improve the quality of dissemination research in the PRC program, the committee recommends that

• **CDC should set specific expectations for dissemination research in the PRC program and encourage the PRCs to communicate their findings concerning dissemination and implementation methods among themselves and to the broader public health community.**

Criteria for Evaluating Prevention Research Centers

The PRCs vary considerably in the extent to which they publish research, disseminate their findings, and interact with local and state programs and agencies. In many of the PRCs there is no clear mechanism to eliminate low-quality projects that are unlikely to yield generalizable or clearly usable results worthy of dissemination through publication. One option for improving the quality assurance procedures at CDC is a modification in the format of the PRCs' annual progress reports. Thus, the committee recommends that

• **CDC should require PRC progress reports to include information on research findings and publications.**

External peer review is a time-tested mechanism for evaluating a research program and identifying areas for improvement. To ensure appropriate scientific review of the PRCs, the committee recommends that

• **An external peer review of each PRC should be conducted in the year prior to the last year of its funding.**

The core funding of the PRCs is dedicated to developing community-based projects that enhance health, build and maintain strong working relationships with community organizations, and establish better-informed public health practice and research communities. In order to set expectations clearly and treat all of the centers fairly, the committee recommends that

• **CDC should establish criteria to evaluate the performance of a PRC over its five-year funding period.**

Funding for the PRC Program

Funding for the PRC program has never equaled the amounts initially authorized by Congress in 1986, and the current inadequate level of funding for PRCs seems to be a critical barrier to the program's long-term success. Thus, the committee recommends that

• **The Congress should increase the appropriation for the core PRC program to the level authorized in PL 98-551 to allow for 13 PRCs to be funded at the $1 million level, as originally intended.**

Peer review has been largely responsible for the remarkable quality, productivity, and originality of U.S. science and technology. In order to ensure the quality and relevance of the research carried out by the PRC program, the committee recommends that

• **Core funding for the PRCs should be determined as a result of open competition, using the peer-review approach that is standard in most federally-funded research programs.**

In the SIP funding mechanism, CDC has found a creative means of supporting PRC research activities beyond the level provided by congressional appropriations. Nevertheless, as a funding mechanism it lacks a systematic approach to setting priorities, calling for proposals, reviewing proposals, and funding the accepted proposals (initial and continuing). Thus, the committee recommends that

- **Priorities for the SIPs should be set through a long-term, interactive process involving the PRCs, CDC, and the public health practice community.**

SIPs have the potential to create innovative opportunities for the PRCs consistent with their themes, but as currently structured, they are more likely to present distractions. By reflecting the capabilities and goals of the PRCs and the PRC program in SIPs, the SIPs are likely to produce innovative research and demonstration projects. Thus, the committee recommends that

- **CDC should assure that the capabilities and goals of the individual PRCs and the PRC program are reflected in the SIPs.**

Another way in which SIPs can advance the science of prevention research is through replication of promising studies in other regions and populations. Therefore, the committee recommends that

- **CDC should make available a portion of SIP funds to encourage collaborative networks, multicenter studies, or replication of promising studies in other regions and populations.**

CDC requires that PRCs use core funds for demonstration projects, collaboration with state and local health (or education) departments, and training, but it does not specify the proportion of funding that should be allocated to each activity. PRCs should have leeway in determining *how* they will achieve core objectives, but should be held accountable for demonstrating that objectives have been achieved. Thus, the committee recommends that

- **CDC should allow the PRCs to determine how to spend their core funds most productively for their varying organizational circumstances.**

SUMMARY AND CONCLUSIONS

By forging links with academia, CDC has created a gateway for access to a cadre of well-trained, university-based researchers who could serve to inform and collaborate with the agency and the public health community regarding health promotion and disease prevention. The PRC program also fosters the development of academic research in questions related to public health practice, community interventions, and the development of community links for translating research findings into practice.

Overall, the committee finds that the PRC has made substantial progress and is to be commended for its accomplishments in advancing the scientific infrastructure in support of disease prevention and health promotion policy, programs, and practices. The committee's review of the efforts of the individual PRCs has indicated that each of the centers has made some contributions toward one or more of the goals of the program, and in the committee's judgment, many of these activities would not have been undertaken in the absence of the PRC program. There are, however, substantial differences among the PRCs in the kinds of activities they have undertaken and the success realized, and only a few centers have made substantial progress on all fronts: research, dissemination, and developing connections with the community and public health practitioners. Given the breadth of the PRC program's goals, the limitations on core funding, and the relative newness of some of the PRCs, the program's successes have been genuine and important.

The committee's review indicates that CDC's management of the program has been creative in the face of limited resources relative to its mandate, dogged in pursuing the mandate over a 10-year period in a bureaucratic environment that was not created or structured for the management of university-based research programs, and skilled in enhancing a sense of community and networking among the funded centers in a time of disappointing funding levels. CDC has fulfilled its initial mandate of "establishing and maintaining centers collaborating through research and demonstration to help fulfill prevention goals consistent with regional and national priorities" (PL 98-551, 1984). By further strengthening the PRC program, the CDC can increase its capacity to contribute to local, state, and national efforts to improve the health of Americans.

1

Introduction

Health promotion and disease prevention are central priorities in the Centers for Disease Control and Prevention (CDC) vision, *Healthy People In A Healthy World Through Prevention* (CDC, n.d.). To advance research in these areas, Congress authorized and the CDC has established a program of university-based Centers for Research and Demonstration of Health Promotion and Disease Prevention. The program is intended to "undertake research and demonstration projects in health promotion, disease prevention, and improved methods of appraising health hazards and risk factors, and shall serve as demonstration sites for the use of new and innovative research in public health technique to improve public health" (PL 98-551). The prevention research centers (PRC) program[3] began in 1986 with funding to three universities. With periodic competitive renewals and expansions of the program, there are now 13 PRCs.[4]

Multidisciplinary faculty at these PRCs, located at schools of public health and academic health centers, focus on a series of related projects on a public health theme defined in terms of special populations, risk factors, or specific health conditions. The PRCs are expected to form partnerships to develop innovative ways to prevent disease and promote health, focus on high-priority

---

[3]Public Law 98-551 created Centers for Research and Demonstration of Health Promotion and Disease Prevention. Throughout this report, the committee refers to these university-based centers as prevention research centers, or PRCs. In referring to the administration of the program by CDC, the committee uses the terminology "the PRC program."

[4]A 14th PRC grant was awarded after the committee completed its final meeting.

innovative ways to prevent disease and promote health, focus on high-priority public health issues, and conduct research and demonstration activities that result in improved public health practice. The PRCs are intended to serve as bridges between science and practice, and from academia to state and local health departments, health care providers and provider organizations, and community organizations, as well as with CDC. Evaluation research is embedded in many of the PRC interventions, the center also train public health professionals in applied prevention research.

Funding for the PRCs includes three components: (1) core center funding from CDC, which must be used, in part, for at least one demonstration project with a state or local health department or board of education; (2) supplemental funding, also from CDC, to address special interest projects (SIPs) proposed annually and funded by various components of CDC each year; and (3) funding from other public and private sources.

HISTORY OF THE PREVENTION
RESEARCH CENTERS PROGRAM

The PRC program was authorized by Congress in 1984 by Public Law 98-551. This legislation was supported by the Association of Schools of Public Health, which viewed the PRC program as a way to enhance health promotion activities by fostering better linkages between the schools of public health and the public health practice community and between academia and CDC. Congress mandated that the PRCs be located at academic health centers capable of providing multidisciplinary faculties with expertise in public health, relationships with professionals in other relevant fields, graduate training and demonstrated curricula in disease prevention, and a capability for residency training in public health or preventive medicine. The PRC program was established at the CDC in 1985, but no funding was appropriated until 1986, when the first three centers were established.

CDC has evolved from an agency born of the need to control malaria in the United States during World War II to the nation's primary agency for the control of a broad spectrum of contemporary health hazards related to environmental and occupational exposures, chronic diseases, and behavioral risks (CDC, 1994). CDC's mission to "promote health and quality of life by preventing disease, injury and disability" (CDC, 1994) and its special relationship with state and local health departments make it a good institutional home for the health promotion and disease prevention content and the community-based focus of the PRC program. Because of the rapidly changing health care environment, CDC sees its role and relationship to the public health community changing significantly with prevention research and dissemination of effective strategies and interventions becoming paramount. To foster the necessary research and development efforts, CDC has sought to develop the capacity to conduct and support prevention research that is recognized as innovative and effective. To address these goals, the scientific research that the CDC supports at academic centers must be innovative and of high quality, and it must include dissemination research and application.

CDC sees the PRC program as (1) providing a sound basis for health promotion and disease prevention and (2) translating research findings into community-based interventions. It identifies four main goals for the program, all intended to help meet national health objectives:

- Maximize resources for complex public health research.
- Make communities accessible and amenable to prevention interventions.
- Increase collaboration among agencies and nontraditional partners.
- Train public health professionals (NCCDPHP, 1996).

GROWTH OF THE PRC PROGRAM

PL 98-551 authorized the Secretary of Health and Human Services to provide funding at the annual level of $1 million per center for a total of 3 centers in 1985, 8 centers in 1986, and 13 centers in 1987. The actual appropriations from Congress, however, have fallen short of these authorized levels. Congress has expanded the PRC program from 3 PRCs and a total budget of $1.5 million to 13 PRCs and a total budget of approximately $7.7 million. This growth is shown in Table 1-1.

In 1993, CDC began providing supplementary funds to the PRCs as a way to increase the levels of research activity within the PRCs through a Special Interest Project (SIP) funding mechanism. The PRCs received a total of $1.3 million through SIP funding in 1993 (ranging from $10,000 to $408,000 per PRC). In 1994 and 1995, the amounts were $3.3 million (ranging from $30,000 to $864,000 per PRC) and $9.5 million (ranging from $82,000 to $1.615 million per PRC), respectively. In 1996, $9.6 million was available for SIPs. Figure 1.1 illustrates the growth of the core funding and SIP components of the PRC program budget.

Most of the PRCs also receive funding from the National Institutes of Health, state health departments, private foundations, and other sources. Some receive additional funding from CDC that is not associated with the PRC program core grants or SIPs. In fiscal year 1996, core funding for the PRC program was about $7.7 million, but CDC estimates that the total funding for

TABLE 1-1 Annual Congressional Funding and Number of PRCs

Year	Core Funding ($ millions)	Number of PRCs	Range of Core Awards Made to each PRC ($ thousands)
1986	1.5	3	406–550
1987	1.6	3	430–579
1988	1.8	5	124–511
1989	2.1	5	187–511
1990	3.8	7	325–650
1991	4.1	7	400–725
1992	5.2	7	420–861
1993	4.8	9	400–581
1994	5.8	12	425–977
1995	7.4	13	360–1,000[a]
1996	7.7	14	n.a.

[a] This represents the PRC program recommendation for funding levels in 1995.

the centers was around $30 million (including SIP funding and nonprogram funding). Some of this additional funding has come to the PRCs as the result of CDC's investment in an infrastructure for prevention research. In addition to the increasing number of PRCs, the program has broadened its geographic distribution and thematic areas. The expansion of the PRC program by geographic areas and thematic interests is shown in Table 1-2.

CDC'S REQUEST FOR A REVIEW OF THE PRC PROGRAM

In 1995, CDC asked the Institute of Medicine (IOM) to review the PRC program to examine the extent to which the program is providing the public health community with workable strategies to address major public health problems in disease prevention and health promotion. IOM established a 10-member committee to evaluate the PRC program. CDC asked the committee to evaluate (1) the overall quality and appropriateness of the health promotion and disease prevention research and demonstration projects being carried out at the PRCs; and (2) CDC's management and oversight of the PRC program. The specific charge to the committee can be found in Appendix B.

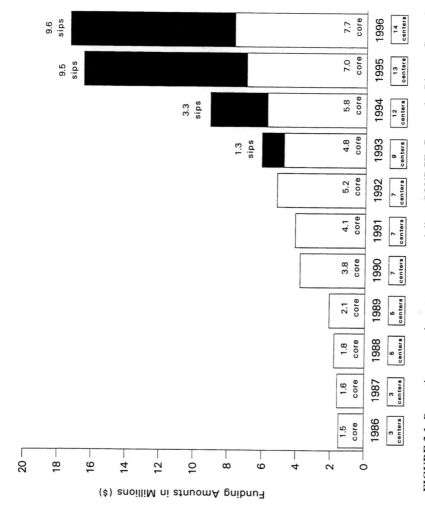

FIGURE 3.1 Prevention research centers program dollars. SOURCE: Centers for Disease Control and Prevention.

TABLE 1.2 Growth of the PRC Program

Year Established	University	Theme
1986	University of North Carolina at Chapel Hill: Schools of Dentistry, Medicine, Nursing, Pharmacy, and Public Health	Workplace health promotion: New approaches to improving worker health
1986	University of Washington, Seattle, School of Public Health and Community Medicine/Group Health Cooperative of Puget Sound	Making prevention work with community partners/ Health promotion in older adults
1986	The University of Texas School of Public Health	From healthy children to healthy adults
1990	Columbia University School of Public Health	Reduction of excess morbidity and mortality in Harlem
1990	The University of Illinois, Chicago, School of Public Health	Health promotion and disease prevention across the lifespan
1993	The University of California at Berkeley School of Public Health	Families, neighborhoods, and communities: A model for action in chronic disease
1993	The University of South Carolina School of Public Health	Promoting health through physical activity
1993	The Johns Hopkins University School of Public Health	Promoting health and preventing disease among urban and rural adolescents
1993	The University of Alabama, Birmingham, School of Public Health	Risk reduction across the lifespan within African-American families
1993	Saint Louis University School of Public Health	Chronic disease prevention in low-income, rural communities
1994	The University of Oklahoma College of Public Health	Health behavior promotion and disease prevention in the Native American population

TABLE 1.2 *Continued*

Year Established	University	Theme
1994	Robert C. Byrd Health Sciences Center of West Virginia University	Risk factors in Appalachia, with emphasis on cardiovascular diseases
1994	University of New Mexico Medical Center	Promoting healthy lifestyles in American Indian families

SOURCE: The CDC Prevention Research Centers Program (D. Labarthe).

Organization of the Study

The committee's report is intended to assist CDC in supporting research in health promotion and disease prevention. The focus of the report is on the roles, functions, plans, actions, and performance of CDC in establishing and maintaining the overall PRC program. The committee's examination of individual PRCs has been for the purpose of understanding the experience and performance of PRCs under varying circumstances of participation, not for the purpose of evaluating the individual PRCs.

The potential of the PRCs to contribute to the fulfillment of the goals of regional and national health promotion and disease prevention was debated, and a decision was rendered in favor of the program when the authorizing legislation was passed. The committee accepts this conclusion without difficulty and without conducting the extensive study that would be required to test the validity or, at this early stage, the achievement of this goal.

As a first step in assessing whether the PRC program is providing the necessary support for the PRCs to perform appropriately and effectively, the committee addressed questions related to the directions the PRCs have staked out for themselves and how the PRC program has provided support for movement in those directions. The committee accomplished this, in part, by examining the circumstances that have allowed some PRCs to flourish in their progress and the circumstances under which other PRCs have waned.

The committee has not assessed the quality of the health promotion and disease prevention research and demonstration projects of individual PRCs. Rather, the focus is on CDC's plans, actions, and support of the overall PRC program to facilitate the appropriate and effective functioning of the PRCs. The research and demonstration projects of the PRCs have been assessed through CDC's two-tiered review process, at the stages of making the initial proposal and reporting annual progress.

Methodology for Reviewing the PRC Program

The committee met three times, in March, May, and July 1996. The PRCs and the CDC provided information about the PRC program to the committee, both at and between the meetings. The committee reviewed documentation about the PRC program, including:

- historic documents about the program, including its legislative history;
- annual funding applications, internal review documents, and peer-review materials about each center;
- applications from centers that did not receive initial or continuing funding;
- criteria given in requests for proposals for new center grants and competitive renewals;
- information about projects receiving SIP funding;
- PRC program vision statements;
- annual reports from each center for each year funding was received.

As a second source of information about the PRC program, the committee developed a questionnaire for the directors of the 13 university-based PRCs. Responses to the questionnaires were followed by scheduled telephone interviews with nine PRC directors, site visits to three PRCs, and a meeting with one PRC director during the committee's July meeting. The telephone interviews, which involved the PRC directors and, quite frequently, key staff, lasted from 90 minutes to 2 hours. Protocols for the interviews and site visits and the questionnaire appear in Appendix C.

The site visits were conducted during a single business day, from 10 a.m. to 4 p.m. The committee selected three PRCs for a site visit based on years of funding, relation to the academic health center, geographical distribution, and population diversity. Site visits were made to one "mature" PRC funded in 1986 (The University of North Carolina), one intermediate PRC funded in 1990 (Columbia University), and a young PRC funded in 1994 (the University of New Mexico). The committee's meeting in July with a PRC director provided an opportunity to hear from a researcher who has been involved with the PRC program since its inception in 1986.[5]

The committee also made one site visit to CDC to conduct discussions with the PRC program staff, as well as CDC staff who work outside the PRC program but who have provided funding to PRCs through SIPs. Committee staff attended the PRC annual meeting in Atlanta in February 1996.

---

[5] One of the committee members also had been a director of one of the first three centers.

OVERALL IMPRESSIONS

By forging links with academia, CDC has created a gateway for access to a cadre of well-trained, university-based researchers who could serve to inform and collaborate with the agency and the public health community regarding health promotion and disease prevention. The PRC program also fosters the development of academic interest in research questions related to public health practice, community interventions, and the development of community links for translating research findings into practice. Overall, the committee finds in this report that CDC has made substantial progress with its PRC program and is to be commended for its accomplishments in advancing the scientific infrastructure in support of disease prevention and health promotion policy, programs, and practices. By further strengthening the PRC program, the CDC can increase its capacity to contribute to local, state, and national efforts to improve the health of Americans.

The PRC program is at a crucial turning point. In Chapter 2 the committee discusses the importance of crafting a vision for the future of the program at this stage in the program's history, and its suggests some elements of a vision for the program. The committee's findings and recommendations appear in chapters 3 and 4. Chapter 3 reviews the research and demonstration projects conducted by the individual PRCs, and Chapter 4 addresses CDC's management and oversight of the program as a whole.

ADDITIONAL PERSPECTIVES ON THE PRC PROGRAM

While the committee was carrying out its work, the PRCs prepared a report that described their progress during the past decade. A summary of the report is in Appendix D. Also during this time, the CDC program staff prepared an information sheet on the program, which is reproduced in Appendix E. The contents of these reports and the perspectives of the PRC directors and the CDC staff were helpful to the committee.

2

A Vision for the Prevention Research Centers Program

THE CHALLENGE AHEAD

The challenges now faced by the PRC program are similar to those faced by universities, especially academic health centers, everywhere in North America. These challenges involve the financial pressures in most of this country's institutions, joined by the need to become visibly contributing partners in their home communities. Universities are being called upon to "reinvent" themselves as close partners with the greater communities they serve. These are opportunities to transform the educational process by using new educational and communication technologies to respond to the unique training and research needs of communities. These challenges suggest an opportunity for the PRC program to place much greater emphasis on its outreach, dissemination, technical assistance, and implementation roles. Collaborative funding of community and state or regional dissemination and implementation efforts must also be pursued so that the responsibility of funding and staffing community, state, and regional programs is shared by all public and private stakeholders—health care providers, public health departments, private businesses, and others. Responding to these challenges, the committee has developed a vision for the PRC program that is described in this chapter. Its purpose is to provide ideas for the PRC leadership as they evolve the system, and to clarify the standard to which the committee held the PRCs and the program as a whole.

Purpose of the PRC Program

The committee's review and discussions with some of those associated with the development of the PRC program indicate that there are at least three ways in which the PRC program can serve CDC's purposes. First, in fulfillment of its mission as the nation's prevention agency, CDC could use the PRC program to undertake the research and development that any successful, forward-looking science-based agency must have. The PRC program could generate new knowledge, from fundamental concepts to practical approaches, and could support prevention practice at CDC, as well as at state and local public health agencies, in communities, and in health service delivery settings. CDC has an organizational focus on community health and has both a unique interest and experience to bring to public health practice research. Increasing numbers of researchers are recognizing the importance of community factors among the determinants of health and the consequent potential for community-based interventions, as well as the value of community involvement in the conduct of health research—that is, setting the research goal or question, developing community-appropriate methodology, interpreting results, and disseminating findings. Through the PRC program, CDC could lead the way in generating needed knowledge about this new community-based approach to research. Although other approaches to health promotion and disease prevention research remain important, addressing community-based interventions would allow CDC to distinguish itself from other research sponsors, develop a promising area of work, and most important, create a field program that reflects the reality of the communities CDC is intended to serve.

Second, CDC could use the PRC program as a way to build capacity for public health practice outside its Atlanta headquarters. The university-based PRCs, which have collaborative relationships with state and local health departments, community organizations, and other entities, might serve as extensions of CDC's activities based in Atlanta and state health departments to field settings that would otherwise be beyond the agency's reach. In this model, the PRCs would function as field laboratories for research and development relevant to CDC's mission and would provide the staff and connections to the community necessary to respond to public health issues that may arise in those communities. More generally, if CDC viewed schools of public health and similar academic institutions as important components of the nation's capacity to address public health problems, a research program could strengthen the institutions, just as National Institutes of Health (NIH) research support since World War II has increased and improved the capacity of American medical schools to address the nation's medical problems (IOM, 1984).

Finally, CDC could use the PRC program as a way to work with disadvantaged communities on critical public health problems. Taking advantage of their locations and the connections that some academic health centers already have with minority communities, CDC-sponsored centers could provide an opportunity to address some of the pressing public health needs of these communities. By focusing its research efforts on issues relevant to particular disadvantaged communities associated with the PRCs, the PRC program could develop new knowledge appropriate to similar communities nationwide.

A Vision for the Future

As any complex program must, the PRC program needs to establish a vision for the future to enable its success as it moves into its second decade. Many options are available. The vision should encourage PRCs, and others who work in health promotion and disease prevention, to expand their activities, moving toward centers characterized by:

- focus on risk conditions and social determinants of health;
- an orientation toward the community;
- interdisciplinarity;
- a means for dissemination research in public health;
- an interactive process for establishing research priorities;
- a role in setting national research priorities.

A Focus on Risk Conditions and Social Determinants of Health

The last several decades have witnessed a resurgence of interest in broader models of health and its determinants, in part as a response to the growing realization that investments in clinical and personal preventive health care were not leading to commensurate gains in the health of populations. McGinnis and Foege (1993) found, for instance, that approximately half of the deaths in the United States were related to behavioral risks. More than half of the recommendations of the U.S. Preventive Services Task Force (1995) dealt with patient counseling interventions to address these behavioral factors. The Lalonde Report introduced a "new perspective" that recognized four elements as critical determinants of health: lifestyles, environment, human biology, and health care organizations (LaLonde, 1974). A broadening interest in health promotion in the United States has been evident in the "Healthy People" initiative since 1979. *Healthy People 2000: National Health Promotion and Disease Prevention Objectives* (USDHHS, 1991) has been officially adopted to guide Public Health Service programs. Unlike the traditional biomedical model that views health as the absence of disease, the new models of health count the presence of good health, full functional capacity, and a positive sense of well-being as outcomes of interest. General factors that affect many diseases or the health of large segments of the population, rather than specific factors accounting for small changes in health at the individual level, are emphasized (Evans and Stoddart, 1994). The new models take a multidisciplinary approach, uniting biomedical sciences, public health, psychology, statistics and epidemiology, economics, sociology, education, and other disciplines.

The importance of considering the origins of health and the underlying risk conditions of disease in individuals and populations is emphasized in these new models. They underscore the interdisciplinary and multisectoral efforts often required to achieve health improvement in communities. Social, environmental, economic, and genetic conditions, in addition to behavioral risk factors, are seen as contributing to differences in health status, and therefore presenting opportunities to intervene.

Through the PRC program, research support and technical assistance can be provided to communities as they strive to improve the health of their populations. Guidance from academia and governmental agencies will be needed to improve the health status of Americans and to achieve healthy communities. The PRC program can play an important role in the adoption of new, broad models for how communities should approach health improvement.

An Orientation Toward the Community

During the decade since the PRC program was begun, there have been substantial changes in the public health establishment's understanding of the importance of the community to the health of the public. Following on *The Future of Public Health* (IOM, 1988), more recent IOM reports (IOM 1996a,b) have stressed the relationship between public health agencies and other community entities and public health's leadership role in improving the community's health. Community health is now seen as a product of many factors, and many segments of the community have the potential to contribute and share responsibility for its protection and improvement. Changes in public policy, in public and private sector roles in health and health care, and in public expectations are presenting both opportunities and challenges for communities as they address health issues.

Contributing to this change of perspective is a wider recognition that health embraces well-being as well as the absence of illness. For both individuals and populations, health can be seen to depend not only on medical care but also on other factors, including individual behavior and genetic makeup and the social and economic conditions affecting individuals and communities. As described by Evans and Stoddart (1994), the multiple determinants of health are best understood in a dynamic relationship, with feedback loops linking social environment, physical environment, genetic endowment, an individual's behavioral and biologic responses, disease, health care, health and function, well-being, and prosperity. This model makes it clear that a wide range of actors, many whose roles are not within the traditional domain of "health activities," both affect and have a stake in a community's health. These include individual health care providers, public health agencies, health care organizations, purchasers of health services, local governments, schools, community organizations, policymakers, and the public.

Because of the importance of the social context in which health-related behavior is determined, community interventions have been the subject of a great deal of interest in the public health community in the last few years. Settings for community interventions include schools, and work sites, as well as whole communities. Approaches to these activities can take passive or active forms. Passive approaches change the physical or social environment and can be oriented toward control by police actions or restriction of substance availability, or toward incentives through taxes, prices, and the like. Active approaches to influence behavior can be targeted directly to individuals through screening and counseling programs, or to groups through the media or educational programs.

Community interventions include, but go beyond, the mass media to include community organization and control. Community interventions also differ in important ways from the medical model; rather than treatment for specific conditions, community interventions focus on knowledge and behavior of individuals and policymakers and aspects of the social and physical environment that influence them. Because of this focus, attitudes and culture as well as personal decisions take on increased prominence. Correspondingly, the science base for community interventions has roots in the social and behavioral sciences as well as in the biomedical sciences. The issue in many cases is not with the evidence of the importance of behavior change, or even the basic social and behavioral science, but with translating this knowledge into action in the community.

As the development of this new understanding about health and the community proceeds, many universities are contemplating major transformations that include forming partnerships with industry, public agencies, and other community organizations to enhance the economic, physical, and social well-being of the institutions, their students, and their surrounding communities. The breakdown of traditional boundaries allows universities to form true partnerships with community organizations for research, service, and teaching activities. The PRCs could serve as leaders in building partnerships, if they are able to progress to a second phase that involves research and dissemination projects that are jointly planned and produced with community partners who have joint ownership of the programs.

Enthusiasm and optimism about getting universities directly involved in the solutions to social problems, however, should not be allowed to overwhelm them with demands beyond their capacities. A major concern is that increased responsibilities may be thrust upon the universities without commensurate increases in resources and that the educational and research missions of the universities will be jeopardized. Even if resources are increased, however, the risk remains that interests and attention of faculty, staff, and students in the universities will be diverted and that dilution of other activities will be inevitable. The PRCs are not intended to substitute for or replace the excellent service implementation partnerships that CDC has with state and local health departments. The PRCs are not intended to substitute for or replace the excellent service implementation partnerships that CDC has with state and local health departments. Public and other social agencies should limit their expectations of the role of universities in directing interventions to ameliorate social ills, and universities should be wisely, if selectively, resolute in resisting both the demands, which are obvious, and the temptations, which may not be.

Interdisciplinarity

Another extension of the conventional research approach is the active and collaborative engagement of multiple disciplines in prevention and health promotion research. This goal cannot be achieved if core faculty from various disciplines pursue separate research agendas on multiple, parallel, discipline-based tracks. A true interdisciplinary approach to research involves the active synthesis of disciplinary perspectives in defining a single research problem, the active merging of methodologies and methods in measuring and analyzing the phenomena under study, and the active reconciliation of multiple levels of analysis in the interpretation of results (Campbell, 1987; Vertinsky and Vertinsky, 1990).

Interdisciplinary research is one of the defining features of *research centers* that distinguishes them from most academic departments and justifies their existence within a university. One view of interdisciplinary research organizations is that their creation depends on uncertainty about a single approach to solve or research the problems they address, and that "a prime danger to the survival of interdisciplinary research organizations (IDROs) stems from strategies initiated by their management to reduce external and internal uncertainties" (Vertinsky and Vertinsky, 1990). The development of an IDRO often depends on identifying an area for research that is important and has been neglected or unsolved by the mainstream disciplines. IDROs that retreat to bureaucratic modes of behavior and specialization to reduce uncertainty or to insure greater security often fall prey to the very limitations of disciplinary departments that justified their creation (Vertinsky and Vertinsky, 1990).

Interdisciplinarity also seeks to consolidate knowledge in ways that are more meaningful to communities' residents and practitioners (Beam, 1982). Public health as an interdisciplinary field has grounded its scientific foundations in epidemiology, biostatistics, social and behavioral sciences, administration, and environmental sciences. Indeed, the development of a cohesive body of knowledge for public health brings together these disciplines in a variety of combinations, depending on the research problem at hand. The development of knowledge in applied fields usually requires some degree of interdisciplinarity (Klein, 1985). This need becomes increasingly clear as emerging health problems are found to be complex, multicausal, and protracted in their duration and their latency period.

A Means for Dissemination Research in Public Health

A systematic, planned approach to dissemination can facilitate the PRCs' integration of research and programs that have been tested or evaluated into practice at the community or clinic level. The CDC has a tradition of working with state health agencies in the prevention of disease and the promotion of health. State and local health agencies play a critical role as linking agents in the process of diffusion of research in public health practice. A recommendation from CDC's First National Conference on Chronic Disease Prevention and Control (CDC, 1987) stated, "if it is true that effective clinical techniques should move quickly to the bedside, it is equally true that new prevention techniques should rapidly reach the community." Prevention centers, in conjunction with state and local health agencies, may enhance that diffusion process.

The universities that provide the institutional base for PRCs can facilitate the dissemination of findings from research and demonstration. This can be accomplished by incorporating research findings into teaching programs, assisting in publication of work in scholarly journals, bringing results to the attention of disciplines beyond public health (e.g., medicine, nursing, social work, pharmacy, and the like), and influencing policymakers. As universities have moved toward more interaction with communities, as is the case among many national and local institutions, they have increased the potential to provide findings to a broad range of community constituencies. They can also generate from their constiutuencies relevant needs and problems deserving exploration in research and demonstration.

An Interactive Process for Establishing Research Priorities

One way to characterize the options facing the PRCs in their relationship to public health practice communities (for example, state and local health departments, nonprofit community organizations, and so on) is as an evolving process for setting research priorities. PRCs adopting this approach must evolve through three steps: (1) the current proactive practice of academically driven research initiatives, (2) a more reactive practice for designing research in response to the needs and input of community agencies, and (3) the development of interactive research practices that involve both academic researchers and the community as equal partners in all phases of a research project.

The interactive model, an ideal to which some PRCs might aspire, focuses on building relationships with communities that represent true partnerships and conducting research that addresses local needs. The current literature refers to the interactive model of applied research as "participatory research" (Fals-Borda and Rahman, 1991; Green et al., 1995) and "empowerment evaluation" (Fetterman, 1994; Fetterman et al., 1995). These are variations on earlier models and traditions of "action research" (Lewin, 1953), "participatory evaluation" (Cousins and Earl, 1995), "developmental evaluation" (Patton, 1994), and "participatory action research" (Park et al., 1993; Whyte, 1991). These approaches to research and evaluation have sought to improve on university-based or even community-based models of research by adding education and action as essential components of the research process. They fit logically and strategically with the legislative mandate of the PRC program and the dissemination and outreach objectives of the PRCs.

A Role in Setting National Research Priorities

National priorities for research are established regularly by federal bodies and agencies. In its allocation of funding to specific research institutes and programs, Congress establishes research priorities. In their selection of specific research initiatives to be included in annual budgets, federal agencies establish research priorities.

Federal agencies tend to establish their priorities for research independently of one another. As a consequence, allocations of interest and resources are quite uneven; some important problems may be neglected altogether because they fall in the bureaucratic cracks between the agencies. It is particularly difficult to bring to bear the resources of funding agencies and research recipients to provide for a concerted and integrated attack on a social problem. We do not, in relation to social problems, have any Manhattan Projects or moon shots.

In health promotion and disease prevention, the lack of coordination in establishing priorities and allocating funds means that problems are almost certain to be attacked piecemeal. The problem of adolescent smoking is unlikely to be dealt with in the context of a broad-scale program of research that should probably include nutrition, exercise, drug and alcohol abuse, dropping out of school, and many other issues. We know that adolescents who have weak attachments to school are more likely to drop out of school, to initiate smoking, to engage in risky sexual behavior, and so on, but we do not know whether increasing their attachment to school would also reduce their risks of other behaviors detrimental to their welfare. It might be that the best way to reduce adolescent smoking or other substance abuse would be to make changes in the educational system (Gerstein and Green, 1993), but under the present system of setting priorities, researchers may never be able to study that idea.

The public health community does not want and probably does not need a single agency to convene and establish higher-level research priorities to direct federal funding decisions. Nevertheless, public health research might benefit a great deal from higher-level multidisciplinary or interdisciplinary groups that would be convened, or otherwise created, to look at health issues in a more comprehensive way, to assemble information that cuts across problem boundaries, and to identify gaps in our knowledge base (Clark and McLeroy, 1995). The PRC program could play a leadership role in encouraging and establishing such groups.

3

The Research and Demonstration Projects Conducted by the Prevention Research Centers

The value of the prevention research center (PRC) program is determined, to a large extent, by the content and the quality of the research and demonstration projects conducted by the individual PRCs. The committee assessed the contribution of the efforts of PRCs in terms of the criteria identified in Appendix B: innovation, methods for project selection, dissemination, incorporation into practice, and balance. The basis for this review, as described in Chapter 1, is written documents from the centers as well as a series of questionnaires, telephone interviews, and site visits.

The committee has not assessed the research and demonstration projects of individual PRCs because the scope of the committee's charge is a review of the entire PRC program, not of the individual centers or their research projects. No comprehensive evaluation of the individual PRCs has ever been done. The committee has examined the range and distribution of performance among the 13 PRCs and the Centers for Disease Control and Prevention's (CDC) oversight of this performance. The PRCs have only recently prepared a unified list of the current projects in each center, so the Committee's review necessarily is qualitative rather than quantitative. A number of specific PRC activities are mentioned in this chapter to illustrate the committee's assessments of the entire PRC portfolio; reference to an activity is not intended to imply endorsements of the activity mentioned.

The committee's findings and recommendations regarding the PRCs themselves, as described in this chapter, indicate general directions for the PRCs, and they may not apply to all centers. Chapter 4 contains recommendations for CDC management and oversight of the PRC program that address some of the issues raised in this chapter.

INNOVATIONS

The first question asked of the committee regards the level of innovation in the research conducted by the PRCs:

• To what extent are the university-initiated research and demonstration projects devoted to new and significant public health issues, new intervention strategies, or new methods to improve the practice of public health?

In addressing this question, the committee found it necessary to expand the traditional criterion of innovativeness to encompass the populations and problems addressed. A research project might not be judged innovative as basic research, but may be innovative in the context of the purpose of the PRC program if it addressed an underserved or previously unreached population, or if it were to test previously tested methods on a different but important health problem.

In these terms, the committee found that the research and demonstration projects conducted by the PRCs were indeed innovative. Nearly every PRC carries out research on underserved populations. These groups include African-Americans, Hispanics, Native Americans, residents of Harlem and Appalachia, adolescents, and elders. Some of the PRCs focus their efforts or individual projects on more specific populations such as rural African-American older adults (South Carolina), public safety personnel (North Carolina), and Korean-American women (Berkeley).

The PRCs have addressed a wide variety of new and important public health problems. Topics that have been or are being addressed by the PRCs include:

• fortification of grains with folates to prevent neural tube defects (Washington);
• perinatal transmission of HIV (Berkeley);
• physical activity and nutrition in pregnancy (South Carolina);
• healthy transition to adolescence (Johns Hopkins);
• reproductive health in manufacturing industries (North Carolina);
• physical activity, estrogen metabolism, and breast cancer risk (South Carolina);
• asthma in African-American and Hispanic communities (Columbia);
• physical functioning and quality of life in older adults (Washington);

• effect of smoking cessation in older adults (Washington).

The PRCs are also effective in applying existing methods to new and important public health problems. Some of the interventions that have been or are being studied at the PRCs include:

• efforts to reduce the risk of perinatal transmission of HIV by improving the quality of education, testing, and counseling services in county prenatal clinics (Berkeley);
• small-group interventions to foster decisionmaking and social skills among 6th grade students who attend school-based health clinics (Johns Hopkins);
• evaluating the impact of educational and enforcement strategies to increase compliance with a new law that prohibits the sales of cigarettes to minors (Columbia);
• school-based health promotion projects that include multicomponent interventions to address sexual risk behavior and violence-related behavior (Texas);
• school-based interventions to improve diet and increase physical activity in elementary school children (Texas);
• culturally specific and sensitive smoking prevention and cessation programs, as well as dietary and exercise programs, for Native American youth (Oklahoma);
• an adolescent pregnancy prevention education program using a computer program called "Babygame" (Columbia);
• counseling to promote consistent condom and spermicide use to reduce STD risk in high-risk women (Alabama);
• a smoking cessation intervention for low-income pregnant women (Texas);
• interventions to control asthma in African-American and Hispanic communities (Columbia);
• workplace health promotion interventions for blue collar women (North Carolina);
• a church-based, volunteer-led community health promotion program for cardiovascular risk factors (Columbia);
• computer-tailored health promotion materials to reduce cardiovascular risk factors in rural primary care settings (St. Louis);
• periodic screening and diabetes prevention programs for Native Americans (Oklahoma);
• program at a rural congregate meal site to improve strength and flexibility of older African-American adults (South Carolina);
• a low-cost, community-based exercise program for elders (Washington);

• a prevention education curriculum for physicians, including both lectures and print material, aimed at increasing physician knowledge of prevention guidelines and the delivery of preventive services to patients (Columbia).

In addition, a number of the PRCs are addressing community interventions for the Women's Health Initiative, led by the National Institutes of Health (NIH), through the Special Interest Project (SIP) program.

Some PRCs have addressed research methodology and the development of new interventions. Some of the best examples include programs to accomplish the following.

• Address problems in survey methods for underserved minority communities, such as inadequate sampling frames, low response rates, lack of telephones, and nonresponse bias (Columbia).
• Develop feasible methods for conducting the Behavioral Risk Factor Surveillance System (BRFSS) in Native American populations (New Mexico).
• Develop community-based measures of environmental and policy factors related to chronic disease risks, as well as intervening variables such as self-efficacy and normative beliefs (St. Louis).
• Create new instruments for the assessment of the health status of older adults (Washington).
• Develop a comprehensive student health survey (Texas).
• Improve statewide surveillance for HIV/AIDS (Berkeley).
• Develop statistical models for cross-validation of structural models for longitudinal studies and for ordinal outcomes for longitudinal clustered designs (Illinois).
• Develop an extensive database on methodology literature and instruments for health promotion research and evaluation in public health (Washington).

Most of the PRCs, however, do not engage in this sort of methodological development. One way to enhance a PRC's ability to develop new research methods is to establish a methodology unit or otherwise identify a group of PRC personnel responsible for methodological development. The PRCs at the University of Illinois and the University of Alabama, Birmingham, for instance, have such units in place. Methodology units of this sort are also likely to increase the PRC's ability to raise research funding from sources other than CDC. Thus, the committee recommends that

• **PRCs should include methodology units or assigned personnel in support of research methods development as a core activity.**

SETTING PRIORITIES IN THE PRCs

Among the questions addressed by the committee were:

• What criteria and methods do—and should—CDC and the universities use to select health promotion and disease prevention research and demonstration projects and to judge their results?

• What is the appropriate balance between research supported by core funding, SIP funding, and other funding; between health promotion research and disease prevention research; and between basic research in health promotion and disease prevention and development of interventions?

Criteria for Project Selection

The establishment of a research center, as opposed to a group of uncoordinated researchers, should have implications for the selection of research topics and the evaluation of their results. One area where the "centerness" of a PRC should be evident is that of project selection, as addressed above. The "centerness" of a program will be reflected more accurately in its structure and the kinds of integrative activities it permits and fosters than in the more obvious ways in which titles and roles are made visible. PRCs will be more effective if they are able to call on the loyalties and participation of their key senior personnel on a frequent and regular basis. Provision for regular staff meetings that are well and willingly attended; frequent occasions for open, shared intellectual interchange; and interlocking collaborative efforts will be more indicative of the existence of a real PRC than any accounting of the sources of compensation or other resources. As a PRC matures, it is to be expected that its senior members will have increasing portions of their time committed to their own projects and to advisory roles in the work of their junior colleagues. As long as their decreasing dependence on center resources is not accompanied by a diminution of interest in the affairs and welfare of the PRC, the center can not only remain intact, but can prosper. Thus, one should expect mature PRCs to show evidence of ongoing programs of an integrative nature and structural arrangements that lead to shared intellectual enterprise and responsibilities.

At the University of Washington, *Healthy People* (USDHEW, 1979) and later *Healthy People 2000* (USDHHS, 1981) have provided guidance for PRC project selection. Columbia University has based its project selection on an analysis of excess mortality and morbidity in Harlem. Projects are chosen jointly with representatives of tribal groups at the University of Oklahoma. Beyond these kinds of examples, however, the committee found little evidence in its interviews, site visits, and record reviews of explicit criteria or systematic methods for selecting research projects in the individual PRCs.

In general, the program of a research center is stronger if it is more than a collection of unrelated projects. With a coherent, coordinated program, for instance, projects can build upon one another's results, and staff gain methodological and substantive expertise that improves the quality of subsequent projects they undertake. The development of such a coherent research program requires careful attention to project selection. Thus, the committee recommends that

- **PRCs should clearly state their criteria for project selection and evaluation.**

Criteria for project selection should be informed by objective data on the importance of health problems, community perceptions, gaps in scientific knowledge, and public health practice needs, as well as the interests and expertise of the PRC. These criteria should include:

- the magnitude of the problem, based on morbidity and mortality data and the number and kinds of people affected;
- the severity of the problem and the effectiveness of available or potential interventions;
- the funding level and degree of activity already present within the community;
- the level of expertise at the PRC;
- public health practice needs;
- the level of interest of local partners and stakeholders.

Stakeholders should be identified and may appropriately include state and local health departments, which have a responsibility to assure that health promotion and disease prevention information and services are available in the community (IOM, 1988, 1996b).

The PRC at the University of Illinois, Chicago, for example, has a portfolio of innovative projects bridging basic and applied research, methodologies, measures, and intervention modalities; multiple channels of communication; multiple behavioral risk factors; and high-risk but underserved populations. This center's framework can be a model for other centers to use in developing a comprehensive, integrated selection of projects (see Box 3-1).

BOX 3.1 Health Promotion and Disease Prevention Research at the University of Illinois, Chicago.

UIC's work bridges five phases of health promotion and disease prevention research (Flay, 1986).

Phase I: Basic, epidemiological, and etiological research as well as theoretical development. UIC researchers have developed a "theory of triadic influence" (Flay and Petraitis, 1994) to unify biological, personality, social, and socioeconomic influences on behavior acquisition and change.

Phase II: Methods development. UIC researchers have emphasized research design, sampling, intervention design, measurement, and statistical analysis. For example, in statistics, UIC researchers have developed new statistical methods and associated computer programs for multilevel analysis of categorical data needed for the analysis of community-level intervention.

Phase III: Efficacy trials of promising interventions. UIC researchers have conducted studies of interventions in the areas of adolescent tobacco use and substance abuse, adult smoking cessation, youth AIDS, and violence. One such project is the Youth AIDS Prevention Program, which integrates school-based human sexuality, drug, STD/HIV/AIDS, and risk reduction education and prevention for junior high and middle-school students with parent and community involvement. This program, tested in 15 ethnically varied Chicago-area school districts in 1991–1993, has been shown to enhance perceived self-efficacy, behavioral intentions, knowledge, and communication skills, as well as attitudes regarding HIV/AIDS. Following eight articles about the program in scientific journals, the program was identified by the DHHS Office of Population Affairs as one of a small number of programs with demonstrated impact on fertility and STD/HIV/AIDS-related risk behaviors.

Phase IV: Studies of the effectiveness of interventions under real-world circumstances. UIC researchers, for example, tested a self-help smoking cessation program incorporating television broadcasting and manuals, and found that it was successful in attracting smokers who were difficult to reach by other means: African-Americans, females, and those with annual incomes under $13,000.

Phase V: Dissemination of interventions. One UIC study examined the dissemination of drug abuse prevention programs in Illinois. Surveys of school administrators, board members, teachers, and parents found that uptake was associated with perceptions about the seriousness of the problem, the acceptance of the program, program effectiveness, and satisfaction with the program.

The community advisory committees that all PRCs are required to have can be helpful in project selection, but their consideration or approval of research projects cannot substitute for explicit criteria and systematic methods. The Johns Hopkins PRC, for instance, has three committees to consult with its constituencies; one with youth; another with community agencies; and a third with academic institutions, national agencies, and the private sector. The PRC advisory committee at the University of Illinois, Chicago, includes leaders in public health, voluntary health agencies, medicine, health media, private industry, and policymaking. The committee suggests that the PRCs ultimately, move toward a fuller collaboration with the community in research, as described in Chapter 2. Systematic procedures and methods for the use of these committees in the project selection and evaluation process are needed by most of the centers.

Quality Control

Given the broad range of research, demonstration, dissemination, and other activities that take place at the PRCs, it is difficult to specify objective measures of the quality of these efforts. The committee's subjective review of the PRC's research portfolios suggests that the quality of research and demonstration projects that are being conducted is highly variable. Some PRCs are conducting extremely high quality research and demonstration projects. In these institutions there tends to be a clear mechanism to eliminate low-quality projects that are unlikely to yield results that can be generalized to other populations, to different health outcomes, and so on.

Most of the PRCs, however, do not seem to have a well-defined process for evaluating the results of their research projects. In general, PRCs describe their projects as relevant to their themes, addressing health problems of importance, or at least acceptable, to the community. The quality of research and demonstration projects may be enhanced by the existence of an internal quality control mechanism for reports, publications, research proposals, and other PRC products. Thus, the committee recommends that

• **PRCs should have an internal quality control mechanism such as a review panel for reports, publications, research proposals, and other PRC products.**

Peer Review

A few PRCs have progressed sufficiently to produce research that has been evaluated by the traditional academic standards of peer review. Peer-reviewed grant applications and publications an important means of reviewing the quality of projects, as well as an important channel for disseminating new knowledge in professional communities. The committee finds that as a group PRCs produce too few peer-reviewed research applications and publications relative to their resources and their maturity; they should be encouraged to pursue research funding through peer review channels other than CDC and to publish their findings in the peer-reviewed literature. Because funding for community-based research is relatively rare, the PRCs should be especially diligent about publishing articles that describe the process and the public health implications of their work in this area. The committee had no objective measure for the evaluation of the quality of non-peer-reviewed products. In this regard, the committee recommends that

• **More of the findings of the PRCs should be published in the peer-reviewed scientific literature.**

Public Health Impact

There are many examples of projects that have had a clear impact on the community's health, as well as policies and practices in public health agencies, health service delivery systems, and other community organizations concerned about public health. This can be seen most plainly through links between the PRCs and community institutions and organizations. The University of Washington PRC's link with the Center for Health Studies at Group Health Cooperative of Puget Sound, for instance, which provides a setting for prevention research as well as a dissemination channel. This PRC also works with local senior centers for dissemination of results on elder health. In New York, Columbia has partnered with the local Safe Kids/Healthy Neighborhoods Coalition. Johns Hopkins is working collaboratively with several local health departments to evaluate teen pregnancy prevention programs and school-based health clinics, and the PRC cooperates with Salisbury State University to improve connections to the rural Eastern Shore region of Maryland. The PRC at the University of North Carolina has worked with local county commissioners and municipal leaders to design strategies for reducing injury rates in their jurisdictions.

The committee's impression, however, is that relatively few of the research efforts have produced impact beyond the immediate community. For instance, new methods for communicating with special target groups like minorities or adolescents developed in one PRC are generally not implemented in other similar groups in other communities. To clarify the impact of the PRC research, the committee recommends that

• **PRCs should document the impact of their activities on public health research, practice, and policy, both locally and nationally.**

In this context and elsewhere in this report, it must be remembered that public health practice involves many public agencies and private community organizations as well as leaders and other individuals in the community (IOM 1988, 1996a, 1996b).

Balance in Research Portfolios

In addressing the question of balance among types of funding and research, the committee found as many different patterns as there were PRCs. Given this experience, it is not possible to make general statements regarding balance that would be appropriate for all centers. Rather, the committee recognizes the need for PRCs' to maintain a coherent program of research, and to be both opportunistic in relation to available funding sources and responsive to emerging community needs. The emphasis on a coherent research theme within a PRC is vital for maximizing the cross-fertilization of ideas and methods and for building on the strengths that the PRC develops over time in a defined area of research. Having a coherent theme is also likely to help a PRC raise research funding from sources other than CDC.

Compared with other research programs in health promotion and disease prevention, the PRC program is unique in its focus on the community. Indeed, the *added value* of the PRC program is its potential for community-based research. This approach to health improvement is relatively new (Patrick and Wickizer, 1995; IOM, 1996b), and carries with it a philosophy and view of the scientific method that encourages the involvement of representatives of residents and practitioners in the communities to be studied, as discussed in Chapter 2. Community-based research of this sort is undertaken as a collaboration in which researchers and community partners participate from the earliest stages of a project, defining research objectives. The involvement of community representatives is evident in all phases of the research—setting goals, selecting and designing methods, and interpreting and disseminating data—and their participation plays a role in maintaining a research focus on issues that are relevant to the community. This approach is viewed by many public health practitioners and applied researchers as a way to facilitate the adoption of new health policies and practices among agencies, professionals, and the public (Green et al., 1995; Park et al., 1994; Schwartz and Capwell, 1995). Given the difficulties of conducting community-based research (Koepsell et al., 1992; Schwartz et al., 1993), there is a special need for CDC to nurture the approach and to discuss it both internally and externally. This approach to research is uncommon among funding agencies, and it is consistent with the organizational goals of CDC regarding a community orientation and commitment to the public health practice community.

Integration of PRC activities with state and local health agencies is a critical as well as explicit component of PRC operations. Involvement of the public health practice community—including state and local public health agencies and community-based organizations, as well as the community or population under study—in the development of their health promotion and disease prevention research agenda should be an important consideration in that agenda-setting process.

CDC has an opportunity to advance the science of community-based research through the PRC program. We use the term "community-based" as defined in Chapter 2 as something more than research on the community, or research in the community. The committee's review of the individual PRCs, indicated that some are more oriented toward the participatory dimensions of this approach than others. Thus, the committee recommends that

• The PRCs should adopt a community-based approach to their research and demonstration efforts.

Toward this end, PRCs could

• involve community representatives in all phases of research and demonstration activities, and study ways to make this involvement most effective;

• pursue research and demonstration projects in which community factors, and community interventions, are paramount;

• develop and improve statistical methods for the evaluation of community-based interventions.

DISSEMINATION AND IMPLEMENTATION ACTIVITIES

The committee was also asked to address the following two sets of questions:

• To what extent are the findings of the research and demonstration projects and related research disseminated?   What methods are used to disseminate the results of the research and demonstration projects?   Are they effective?

• To what extent are the findings of research and demonstration projects incorporated into prevention practice, particularly by state and local health departments?

A major focus of the PRCs is the dissemination of their research findings and products to the public health practice community. Achieving changes in individual behavior and public health practices requires varying approaches. Some populations will, by reason of their special characteristics, require unusual efforts and considerable innovativeness.   Improving dissemination and implementation practices calls for research that will inform health promotion professionals, educators, and policymakers about the most appropriate methods for disseminating health messages among different populations.

The PRCs have employed a variety of methods for dissemination, including publishing in the scientific literature; providing workshop-mediated training methods; using advanced communications technologies, including interactive media; developing written and graphic materials for lay audiences; distributing training materials for professional and varied lay audiences; and attending meetings to present results to a wide variety of audiences (for example, local and state health departments, policymakers, public health professionals, lay audiences, education and social science professionals, and numerous organizations including schools, work sites, managed care organizations, and voluntary health organizations). These communications have involved materials to enhance awareness, information of a cognitive nature, and activities devised to improve performance skills.

Some specific examples of PRC dissemination efforts are as follows:

• a summer institute for public health practitioners from HMOs, work sites, hospitals, and health departments (Washington);

• teleconferences to a rural collaborating center (Johns Hopkins);

• workshops for state and local health departments on best practices in adolescent health (Johns Hopkins);

• publication of "policy news briefs" that describe national policies and legislation related to children and adolescents, "issue briefs" that summarize major research findings, newsletters about the center's activities, and "Health of Maryland's Adolescents," a fact book with health, education, and social indicators on adolescents (Johns Hopkins).

• electronic bulletin boards (South Carolina).

The dissemination and implementation activities among the PRCs tend to have three elements: (1) conveying information to appropriate audiences; (2) developing methods for incorporating information into public health practice; and (3) evaluating the effectiveness of the attempts to influence public health practice and improve understanding of the entire dissemination process.

The PRCs differ in both the effort they devote to dissemination and implementation and the nature of those efforts. Some PRCs do not appear to place a high priority on dissemination and implementation, some have ambitious plans that are not being carried out because of reductions in CDC funding levels, and some PRCs have experience and expertise in such activities.

Some of the dissemination efforts of PRCs have been innovative and deserving of emulation and further testing. Examples of such efforts include bumper stickers devised by children from the local community, which are thought to be especially commanding of attention; activation of a lay group to bring political pressure to bear to maintain health promotion efforts for their group; and development of a game for adolescents devised to increase their understanding of critical issues related to their health.

On the whole, however, the committee found that relatively little effort was expended in dissemination activities in the majority of PRCs. Indeed, the committee found that many PRCs are in an early stage of development. During this early phase, PRCs must devote a large proportion of their core funding to establishing a research program. PRCs can expend core funds justifiably to help initiate a cohesive program of research, but such research should then be continued through regular research funding channels so that an adequate proportion of core funds can be devoted increasingly to outreach and technical assistance activities.

Research findings and products from the PRCs and CDC should be disseminated to all PRCs, their communities, and their regional populations; to the research and professional communities through scientific and professional literature; and to the public health practice community and the general public. Thus, the committee recommends that

• **The PRC program, as a whole, should increase its focus on dissemination efforts.**

PRCs can employ a variety of methods for dissemination, as illustrated above, including publishing in the scientific literature; providing workshop-mediated training methods; using advanced communications technologies, including interactive media; developing written and graphic materials for lay audiences; and distributing training materials for professional and varied lay audiences. PRC personnel can also attend meetings to present results to a wide variety of audiences (for example, local and state health departments, policymakers, public health professionals, lay audiences, education and social science professionals, and numerous organizations including schools, work sites, managed care organizations, and voluntary health organizations). These communications should involve materials to enhance awareness, information of a cognitive nature and activities devised to improve performance skills.

Prevention Networks

The impact of the PRC program can be enhanced through cooperative dissemination activities among the PRCs, and between the network of PRCs and other health promotion organizations such as state and local health departments in the United States and elsewhere. Dissemination activities, especially those involving the academic and public health practice communities jointly, can accelerate the diffusion of new public health practices (Schwartz and Capwell, 1995). The PRCs can encourage these activities by taking the lead in creating a national network for dissemination. These efforts should involve the use of advanced communication technologies. Thus, the committee recommends that

• **PRCs should seek to be part of regional and national networks for prevention that include CDC, the public health practice community, and other relevant parties.**

Dissemination Research

It is important to distinguish between dissemination activities and research on dissemination. The goals of *dissemination* are to (1) convey information regarding effective prevention programs to public health officials, other health professionals, and community leaders and (2) inform the public about health-related matters. *Dissemination research*, on the other hand, seeks to identify better ways to communicate information to the public and to practitioners. The Texas PRC, for instance, has conducted dissemination research to demonstrate the effectiveness of interventions designed to influence schools to adopt effective tobacco prevention programs.

In reviewing the activities of the PRCs, the committee found many instances of dissemination activities, but few projects focused on dissemination research. Since the university-based PRCs are attempting an array of dissemination approaches with a wide range of public and professional audiences, and because academic institutions have some research capacity, they are in a unique position to carry out dissemination research. Thus, the committee recommends that

- **The PRCs should increase their dissemination *research* efforts.**

SUMMARY AND CONCLUSIONS

By forging links with academia, CDC has created a gateway for access to a cadre of well-trained, university-based researchers who could serve to inform and collaborate with the agency and the public health community regarding health promotion and disease prevention. The PRC program also fosters the development of academic research in questions related to public health practice, community interventions, and the development of community links for translating research findings into practice.

Overall, the committee finds that the PRC program has made substantial progress and is to be commended for its accomplishments in advancing the scientific infrastructure in support of disease prevention and health promotion policy, programs, and practices. By further strengthening the PRC program, the CDC can increase its capacity to contribute to local, state, and national efforts to improve the health of Americans. The committee's review of the efforts of the individual PRCs has indicated that each of the centers has made some contributions toward one or more of the goals of the program, and in the committee's judgment many of these activities would not have been undertaken in the absence of the PRC program. There are, however, substantial differences among the PRCs in the kinds of activities they have undertaken and their success, and only a few centers have made substantial progress on all fronts: research, dissemination, and developing connections with the community and public health practitioners. Given the breadth of the PRC program's goals, the limitations on core funding, and the relative newness of some of the PRCs, the program's successes have been genuine and important.

4

Management and Oversight of the Prevention Research Centers Program

In this chapter the committee presents its findings and recommendations regarding the management and oversight of the prevention research centers (PRC) program. The discussion focuses on management issues that are related to the quality of the research and demonstration projects undertaken by the individual PRCs, as discussed in the preceding chapter. These issues include the definition of prevention research, criteria for evaluating the PRCs, and procedures for mobilizing and allocating resources in their support. The committee also addresses the degree to which effective collaboration is occurring between PRCs and their communities, among the PRCs as a network, and beyond the PRCs to the national and international community of researchers, policymakers, planners, and practitioners in disease prevention and health promotion. The recommendations in this chapter suggest ways that CDC can help the center program evolve in the directions identified in chapter 2.

VISION AND GOALS

As an agency, the Centers for Disease Control and Prevention (CDC) focuses on public health practice rather than funding university-based research. Nevertheless, through its interviews and site visits, the committee found that the adoption and integration of the PRC program by CDC has been relatively smooth. Through their research and demonstration activities, the PRCs can make—and have made—significant contributions toward meeting some of the national goals and objectives of *Healthy People 2000* (USDHHS, 1991),

49

Whether CDC as a whole has recognized this asset is unclear. CDC's strategic plan (CDC, 1994) makes mention of the PRC program, but it does not appear to feature the program as a resource.

As it recreates its vision for the future, CDC should consider the important and changing relationships between communities and universities discussed in Chapter 2. To ensure that the PRC program remains relevant to critical current public health issues, the committee recommends that

• **CDC should ensure that the vision and goals of the PRC program are compatible, mutually supportive, and consistent with the agency's overall strategic plan and with *Healthy People 2000*. The PRC program's vision and goals should define, in a clear and comprehensive way, the contributions of the PRC program to national priorities.**

A strategic plan, developed collaboratively by the CDC staff and the PRC directors, might help to clarify the program's actual and potential contributions.

Prevention Research

CDC defines prevention research in the application guidelines for the PRC program as research designed "to yield results *directly applicable* to interventions to prevent occurrence of disease and disability, or the progression of detectable but asymptomatic disease". In the context of the broad spectrum of research defined by the National Institutes of Health (NIH) (Moskowitz, et al., 1981), CDC has described the research conducted under its PRC program as applied research. The definition, however, should not be interpreted as limiting the scope of research to disease prevention priorities, as it sometimes appears to do in CDC documents—it should include health promotion. Health promotion requires a scope of research that may not have a *direct* application to prevention of specific diseases or disabilities, at least in the short run. Health promotion research, for instance, addresses risk-taking among adolescents, which indirectly affects lifelong patterns of tobacco, alcohol, and substance use, as well as sexual behaviors that affect teen pregnancy, sexually transmitted diseases, and AIDS. At least three of the PRCs (Hopkins, Illinois, and Texas) are addressing these issues. Health promotion research, generally encompasses the examination of underlying *risk conditions,* which may not have an immediate influence on the incidence of diseases and disability, as well as more proximal *risk factors.* Health promotion research also includes the examination of processes that build the understanding and skills, mobilize the resources, and reinforce the actions of individuals and communities to cultivate health and to improve the quality of life. In order for the PRC program to remain consistent with current theory and practice in health promotion and disease prevention, the committee recommends that

- **CDC should modify its definition of *prevention research* as articulated in the application guidelines for the PRC program to encompass the broader scope of health promotion research needed to address the underlying determinants of health (risk conditions) and to build the capacity of individuals and communities to "cultivate health," rather than to focus solely on those determinants with immediate application to disease prevention (risk factors).**

THEMATIC FOCUS

In the committee's experience, as discussed in chapter 2, academic centers are more likely to build a cohesive program of research and to have a major impact on public health problems when the center develops a strong sense of its own identity. Integrating major research projects around a common theme is one of the best ways to build and maintain cohesiveness and continuity. Such an approach requires strategic planning for each five-year period of core funding and involves putting proposed efforts into research that is most reflective of a center's unique identity.

CDC requires that each PRC adopt a thematic focus for its research and demonstration efforts. A theme is a useful concept for defining a PRC's central mission and its priorities in health promotion and disease prevention. Over time a center's identity can adapt in response to both internal initiatives and external needs. An example of such an approach is the University of Washington's original theme of elder health which later evolved into an additional theme of health for the disabled. Reactively responding to the multiple research topics of the Special Interest Projects (SIPs) can take a center in many directions at once, resulting in fragmentation rather than integration, and diminished focus on in-depth research that ultimately may have the greatest impact on the health of the community.

PRCs, however, are faced with a dynamic tension between criteria based on their themes and those defined by the SIP program and other funding opportunities. Beginning in 1993, CDC has made supplementary funding available to PRCs through this mechanism, in which research topics are identified (and funds provided) by CDC program units, and only PRCs are eligible to compete for the funds. Current planning for SIP funding has been an ad hoc process of garnering funds remaining at end of the fiscal year from agencies, divisions, or offices of the federal government that can use the SIP funding mechanism to expedite spending for discrete research projects.

Although the funding occurs in an expedient way, less encumbered by bureaucratic requirements than other means of government procurement, it has the disadvantage of being hurried and is an unstable funding mechanism. In addition, some of the PRC researchers have raised questions about the process of developing research topics and whether there is sufficient input from the research community and other experts in the public health practice community outside CDC. The resulting topics may not reflect state-of-the-art approaches to research. While SIPs have the potential to create innovative opportunities for the PRCs consistent with their themes, they also have the potential to present distractions from thematic research agendas. If the PRCs are to make progress in their self-identified thematic areas, they need to have a long-term commitment to a focused research agenda.

Based on its interviews and document review, the committee finds that investigator-initiated research tends to be driven by PRC themes and demonstrates commitment to a focused research agenda, whereas SIP-initiated research is generally driven by CDC's internal interests and short-term needs. Although some SIPs have a clear association with the goals of the PRC program as a whole and the strengths and themes of some PRCs, others do not. PRC program staff at CDC need to address the disjoint between PRCs' themes and CDC's internal interests and short-term needs.

It appears that CDC has not communicated whether themes should be paramount in the selection of projects. Guidance from CDC that clarifies the role of PRC themes in selecting projects would be beneficial to the PRCs. In addition, CDC has not specified whether it has expectations about progress toward national goals in the thematic areas, and if it does, the potential roles of the PRCs in achieving these goals. The guidance provided by CDC should be relevant to the selection of investigator-initiated core projects as well as SIPs. In order to clarify CDC's expectations regarding the PRC program's contributions, the committee recommends that

• **CDC should provide guidance to the PRCs about the role of the PRCs' themes in selecting core research and demonstration projects and SIPs.**

NETWORKING, COMMUNICATION, AND DISSEMINATION

Improved Communication and Interaction

The PRC program has created a group of 13 PRCs with similar interests and goals. Several share a focus on similar health problems or populations. No individual PRC has the capacity, interest, or resources to cover the full range of research, from epidemiologic research to research that assesses interventions at the community level and the dissemination and implementation of effective interventions across communities. Collectively, however, the PRCs have this capacity, which is necessary to reach the goals of the PRC program. The groups of researchers, their community constituents, and the circle of public health practitioners who collaborate in the PRCs' activities comprise a valuable network for exchanging ideas, disseminating results, and generating new projects. CDC serves as the fulcrum for networking and communication. Two of the recent SIP initiatives from CDC (on tobacco and adolescent health) have encouraged networking among the PRCs on specific issues.

The committee's review has suggested that the interaction between the PRC program staff at CDC and the individual PRCs has realized some success in linking the efforts of the 13 PRCs. The tobacco network funded by a SIP initiative is an excellent example. Nevertheless, the links among PRCs and between an individual PRC and PRC program staff at CDC and/or other CDC efforts can be improved. In general, projects encouraged by PRC program staff at CDC are not always focused on topics that address the PRCs' central interests and capabilities. This can be attributed to some degree to a lack of communication between PRC program staff at CDC and other CDC units, as well as a lack of opportunity to identify mutually beneficial and innovative projects.

The PRC program can enhance prevention research and the public's health through improved communication and networking mechanisms. To achieve this goal, each PRC should be called upon periodically to report on new knowledge gained that warrants replication or adaptation and evaluation in other PRCs that serve different populations. While some PRCs have generated interesting and significant findings, innovative research and demonstration projects have generally not been replicated within the PRC network. Annual reports to CDC describe activities that PRCs undertake, but not the lessons learned. They are therefore not a source of information that would allow individual PRCs, the PRCs as a group, or the PRC program staff at CDC to build on their own efforts. CDC should encourage the replication of promising studies at other PRCs (Campbell, 1987). The annual meetings provide an opportunity for the PRCs to discuss findings and their appropriateness for replication, multicenter trial, or broad dissemination to the public health practice community. In order to consolidate the information for public health policy being gained from the PRC program, the committee recommends that

• **CDC should provide more opportunities for the PRCs to meet collectively, share lessons learned, exchange information related to findings, activate their collective communication channels on behalf of worthy**

projects, and provide mutual support, especially from strong PRCs to fledgling centers.

CDC efforts to this end could include:

• providing resources for periodic meetings of the PRCs' staff at both senior and junior levels for substantive discussion of research issues through presentation of papers, discussion of methods, planning for collaborative projects, and the like;
• using national meetings, such as the American Public Health Association's annual meeting, to promote communication among PRCs and to reach the broader public health constituency;
• continued development of means for electronic communications among the centers using the Internet and the World Wide Web;
• developing mechanisms to involve individual PRC investigators in decisions related to SIPs and other special projects, strategies for dissemination of research results, and promising new research directions.

Community Input

The added value of the PRC program is its focus on community-based research, and CDC should encourage the public health practice community and other agencies and sectors to take greater advantage of the resource represented by the PRCs in their region and elsewhere. Another way for CDC to achieve greater involvement of the PRCs with the practice community would be to require, as a condition of funding, that the planning processes at PRCs involve representatives from their communities. This would be consistent with the funding conditions that CDC places on state and local health departments. The currently mandated community advisory boards are a step in this direction, but they do not seen to be effective in developing the kind of dialog between the PRCs and their communities called for in Chapter 2. Thus, to foster better connections between the PRCs and the communities they work with, the committee recommends that

• **CDC should develop strategies for improving community input into the PRCs.**

Dissemination Research

As discussed in Chapter 3, the overall amount of *research* on dissemination and implementation appears to be very limited, whether viewed within individual PRCs or across the entire PRC program. PRCs have not exchanged information in a systematic way, and opportunities for replication of investigations into dissemination and implementation have not been exploited. PRCs have not regularly and systematically reported their findings concerning dissemination and implementation to CDC, and CDC does not have a mechanism for assembling findings from the PRCs in order to promote such activities. Thus, to improve the quality of dissemination research in the PRC program, the committee recommends that

• **CDC should set specific expectations for dissemination research in the PRC program and encourage the PRCs to communicate their findings concerning dissemination and implementation methods among themselves and to the broader public health community.**

CRITERIA FOR EVALUATING PRCs

The PRCs vary considerably in the extent to which they publish research, disseminate their findings, and interact with local and state programs and agencies. Based on its interviews, site visits, and document reviews, the committee believes that this is because CDC has not established clear expectations for the PRCs. In fact, CDC does not require that the PRC's results be evaluated, except in funding renewal applications, and no comprehensive evaluation of the individual PRCs has ever been done. The PRC program staff at CDC should, in consultation with the PRCs, set explicit performance expectations and establish a mechanism for periodic evaluation of the PRCs. In this way, CDC can influence the PRCs' output toward high achievements while avoiding micromanagement.

The committee reviewed the quality of the PRCs' research and demonstration projects using standard academic criteria (peer-reviewed publications) and found that the quality of the PRCs' research and demonstration projects is highly variable. In many of the PRCs there is no clear mechanism to eliminate low-quality projects that are unlikely to yield generalizable or clearly usable results worthy of dissemination through publication. A few PRCs produce research that consistently meets the traditional academic standards, but these PRCs are in the minority. Overall, the PRCs produce too few peer-reviewed research publications relative to the resources available and the life span of the PRCs. The committee recognizes that the PRCs make other contributions to health promotion and disease prevention research, and does not believe that academic criteria should dominate the evaluation of the PRCs, but it had no objective or independent measure for the evaluation of the quality of non-peer-reviewed products.

Progress Reports

One option for improving the quality assurance procedures at CDC is a modification in the format of the PRCs' annual progress reports. At present, the annual progress reports do not include measures of project results such as data gathered and their importance and summaries of publications. Instead, they offer measures of what has been done such as meetings attended, and data collected. The annual progress report would be a better quality assurance tool if it contained both results and process measures. Thus, the committee recommends that

• **CDC should require PRC progress reports to include information on research findings and publications.**

Peer Review

There is currently no requirement for external peer review of PRCs. Only applicants for new grants and competitive renewals receive external reviews as part of the application process. External peer review is a time-tested mechanism for evaluating a research program and identifying areas for improvement, and it can help a research program to overcome obstacles to success. Ideally, the external peer review should consist of a review of publications and other PRC products along with a site visit. External peer review should occur sufficiently far ahead of an application for refunding to allow time to make needed changes, at the same time that it assists CDC in forming the basis of its eventual decision about renewal of a PRC (i.e., at least one year ahead of the refunding application). To ensure appropriate scientific review of the PRCs, the committee recommends that

• **An external peer review of each PRC should be conducted in the year prior to the last year of its funding.**

The core funding of the PRCs is dedicated to developing community-based projects that enhance health, building and maintaining strong working relationships with community organizations, and establishing better-informed public health practice and research communities. PRCs must demonstrate that they have used core funding successfully. The measures of success include demonstration programs, productive working relationships with community institutions, and dissemination of research findings. Most centers use core funding to enhance their capacity to do high-quality, investigator-initiated research and carry out community-based interventions. A key measure of success, therefore, is the amount of funds raised to support these projects. In order to set expectations clearly and treat all of the centers fairly, the committee recommends that

- **CDC should establish criteria to evaluate the performance of a PRC over its five-year funding period.**

The criteria should enable one to measure performance in the following programmatic areas:

- development of innovative research and demonstration projects;
- success in conducting demonstration projects (the extent of implementation, proper evaluation, effective dissemination of research findings and lessons learned, altered health behaviors, practitioner functioning, program planning, policy decisionmaking in the population, and other measures);
- publication of research articles in peer-reviewed journals;
- other peer-reviewed products such as videotapes, curriculum, and intervention program guidelines that communicate research results to public health practitioners and the population that they serve;
- an effective working relationship with the public health practice community, including but not limited to official state and local health departments;
- success in disseminating research results to public health practitioners in the PRC's local area and elsewhere;
- a demonstrated role in enhancing public health resources in the community (measured by the number of trainees placed in local public health agencies, the impact on policy changes in the community, and similar activities);
- measures of sustained impact on the community, state, or nation;
- success in competing for other funding, including SIPs, foundation support, community and state funds, and federal grants.

FUNDING FOR THE PRC PROGRAM

Core Funding

Perhaps the most consistent message the committee received from the PRCs was their great need for stable core funding and the perceived inadequacy of the level of core funding provided by CDC. Neither the funding level for individual PRCs nor the overall PRC program has ever equaled the amounts initially authorized by Congress in 1986. In several instances, the PRCs have been unable to pursue dissemination and evaluation activities for lack of adequate funding.

The inadequate level of funding for PRCs seems to be a critical barrier to the program's long-term success. When CDC reduces awards from the proposed level, PRCs are unable to accomplish all the work originally planned. Dissemination and implementation efforts tend to be costly and labor-intensive, and are thus likely to be diminished in scope and intensity in response to reduced funding. Yet these are very important facets of PRC activities. These reductions in funding levels by CDC have adversely affected the quality of the PRCs' dissemination research, as well as the sharing of information between PRCs and the broader public health community. Green and Kreuter (1991) document this "poverty cycle" in the field of health education, and indicate how it can be overcome.

The committee supports CDC's commitment to providing core funds on an ongoing basis to allow PRCs to undertake innovative community-based research activities that are difficult, if not impossible, to support through other funding sources. The committee emphasizes, however, that the CDC needs to encourage the use of core funding to support activities that are likely to produce generalizable research results that will advance the science of health promotion and disease prevention. Thus, the committee recommends that

• **The Congress should increase the appropriation for the core PRC program to the level authorized in PL 98-551 to allow for 13 PRCs to be funded at the $1 million level, as originally intended.**

The committee believes that range of core activities expected of the PRCs (as described elsewhere in this chapter), especially given increased costs in the last decade, fully justifies a core funding level of $1 million per center, as originally authorized. The committee does not have enough information on the budgets of the individual centers, or the effectiveness of the the projects supported by core funds, to make any more specific funding recommendation.

Open Competition

One of the hallmarks of the U.S. research and development system since World War II has been the involvement of nongovernment scientists in setting the detailed scientific agenda of federal research agencies. Part of the social contract between science and government is that scientists should play major roles in providing advice about the scientific agenda, while policymakers should set broad strategic goals and provide the resources needed to reach them. This approach, implemented most clearly in the peer-review process of the National Science Foundation and the National Institutes of Health, is seen as one of the most important reasons that these agencies have been successful in harnessing scientific research to meet national needs in the last half-century. Reviewing this experience in the context of improving the process of allocating federal funds for science and technology, a recent National Academy of Sciences report (NAS, 1995) states that "because competition for funding is vital to maintain the high quality of [federal science and technology] programs, competitive merit review, especially that involving external reviewers, should be the preferred way to make awards."

The NAS report relies on the principle that the highest-quality projects and people should be supported with federal research funds, and finds that the best-known mechanism to accomplish this is some form of open competition involving evaluation of merit by peers. Competitive merit review requires the use of criteria that include technical quality, the qualifications of the proposer, relevance and educational impacts of the proposed project, and other factors pertaining to research goals rather than to political or other nonresearch considerations. Open competition means that, at some level within the framework of an agency's mission, researchers propose their best ideas and anyone may apply and be funded, regardless of institution or geographic location. In the case of highly targeted missions, however, quality can also be maintained by knowledgeable program managers who have established external scientific and technical advisory groups to help assess quality and to help monitor whether agency needs are met.

The committee agrees that merit review—which emphasizes competition among ideas, diversity of funders and performers of research and development, and organizational flexibility—has been largely responsible for the remarkable quality, productivity, and originality of U.S. science and technology in the past. The PRC program was established to improve the capacity of schools of public health and academic health centers to conduct research that can be applied to public health practice, and this goal is to be lauded. This aim should be preserved, and high-quality research should not be hampered by restrictive application criteria.

To further these aims, competition for PRC grants should focus on public health researchers, and CDC should be particularly responsive to applicants who demonstrate a capacity for multidisciplinary approaches to public health problems. Competition for PRCs should not be restricted to a single state; this is unnecessarily restrictive. The network of PRCs should strive to be a national resource that is responsive to all states and territories and that funds the most qualified research proposals. Thus, in summary, the committee recommends that

• **Core funding for the PRCs should be determined as a result of open competition, using the peer-review approach that is standard in most federally-funded research programs.**

Special Interest Projects

In 1993, CDC began providing supplementary funds to the PRCs through a Special Interest Project (SIP) funding mechanism as a way to increase the levels of research activity within the PRCs, and simultaneously address CDC research needs. In 1995, PRCs received $9.5 million (ranging from $82,000 to $1.615 million per PRC) under this program, more than the total core funding. Funding for the community intervention portion of the NIH Women's Health Initiative recently has been channeled through the SIP program.

In this funding mechanism, CDC has found a creative means of supporting PRC research activities beyond the level provided by congressional appropriations. The program also provides a simple means (in an agency not set up to fund research, as NIH is) for CDC units to fund university-based research to meet program needs. As a funding mechanism, however, it lacks a systematic approach to setting priorities, calling for proposals, reviewing proposals, and funding the accepted proposals (initial and continuing). To date, planning for SIP funding has been an ad hoc process of garnering funds at the end of the fiscal year from agencies, divisions, or offices of the federal government that use the SIP funding mechanism to expedite spending to complete discrete research projects. Although the funding is accomplished in an expedient manner, less encumbered than other means of government procurement by bureaucratic requirements that are inappropriate for a research program, it is neither a satisfactory nor a stable means of funding research. It tends to be rushed, confusing for those responding to the requests for applications (RFAs), and frustrating to funders when the responses to RFAs are insufficient. In addition, the process of developing research topics tends to be completed without the benefit of input from the research community and other experts in the public health practice community outside CDC. The resulting topics often do not reflect state-of-the-art approaches to research.

The committee encourages CDC to promote innovation by developing a process of research formulation that is more interactive than either the proactive process of most SIP funding or the reactive process of investigator-initiated grants that have not included consultation with either local or federal consumers of research. One option would be for CDC to institutionalize a triangulation process that would involve PRCs, state or local health departments, and CDC in a process of developing research topics. Thus, the committee recommends that

- **Priorities for the Special Interest Projects (SIPs) should be set through a long-term, interactive process involving the PRCs, CDC, and the public health practice community.**

SIPs have the potential to create innovative opportunities for the PRCs that are consistent with their themes, but as currently structured, they are more likely to present distractions. By reflecting the capabilities and goals of the PRCs and the PRC program in SIPs, the SIPs are likely to produce innovative research and demonstration projects. Thus, the committee recommends that

- **CDC should assure that the capabilities and goals of the individual PRCs and the PRC program are reflected in the SIPs.**

One of the most successful SIPs is a tobacco network project, which provided a small amount of funding to 10 PRCs to develop a collaborating network of projects. This SIP should be used as a model for developing other networking SIPs. Another way in which SIPs can advance the science of prevention research is through replication of promising studies in other regions and populations. Therefore, the committee recommends that

- **CDC should make available a portion of SIP funds to encourage collaborative networks, multicenter studies, or replication of promising studies in other regions and populations.**

CDC assigns a staff liaison to each SIP project funded at a PRC, including projects funded under the NIH Women's Health Initiative. These assignments are made to provide guidance to the PRC researchers and to ensure that the funding unit's program goals are addressed. In some cases, the PRC staff are not experienced in the relevant research areas, and the assignment of a liaison is beneficial. In other cases, however, the university-based researchers are more knowledgeable about a subject area than the CDC staff. If CDC feels that the assignment of liaisons to all SIP projects must continue, the purpose should be clarified, and liaisons used to help create integrated networks, as discussed above.

Allocation of Core Funds

CDC requires that PRCs use core funds for demonstration projects, collaboration with state and local health (or education) departments, and training, but it does not specify the proportion of funding that should be allocated to each activity. PRCs can expend core funds justifiably to help initiate a cohesive program of research, but such research should then be continued through regular research funding channels so that an adequate proportion of core funds can be devoted increasingly to outreach and technical assistance activities. The committee considered varying formulas for proportionate allocation and earmarking of PRCs' core funds for purposes of infrastructure support, research activity, and dissemination and evaluation functions. It concluded that the levels of development and other resources available to the PRCs vary so widely that any single prescription for the allocation of core funds would be inappropriate for some centers, and potentially counterproductive for others.

This should not be interpreted as a recommendation for less oversight by CDC; the intent of the recommendation is to allow flexibility regarding the percentage of funds allocated across mandatory core activities. PRCs should have leeway in determining *how* they will achieve core objectives, but should be held accountable for demonstrating that objectives have been achieved. Thus, the committee recommends that

• **CDC should allow the PRCs to determine how to spend their core funds most productively for their varying organizational circumstances.**

CDC, no doubt, wishes to attract strong, research-oriented institutions that will add to the nation's understanding of prevention and health promotion, work with communities, and disseminate promising results. There are several, somewhat obvious, benefits to an institution that becomes a PRC. For example, the program ensures the availability of funds that will remain reasonably stable over five years and offers the potential to leverage new funds, especially through access to the SIPs. Nevertheless, there are potential drawbacks to the PRC program that may cause hesitation or a decision not to compete. Consideration of these may suggest ways for CDC to strengthen the program.

For some institutions, the amount of core funding available may not be adequate to cover the considerable amount of faculty and staff time needed to initiate and maintain a PRC. Faculty diverted from teaching or from research projects with larger budgets may generate costs not fully covered by core funds.

In addition, much health-related research is funded by agencies that are not primarily interested in community-focused research emphasizing collaboration and, a PRC may not be the best mechanism for leveraging other large, non-CDC, grant support. Further, the process of formulating SIPs appears to exclude academia; that is, CDC determines the priorities, and these may not be central to the primary interests of a given PRC. The attraction of applying for SIPs could thus be diminished because a PRC may not be successful, and securing a SIP may divert faculty from the major work of the PRC.

Many institutions, especially schools of public health, are interested in developing their ability to link with communities and engage in more participatory, partnership-oriented research. Creating and maintaining the interface and capacity for these activities is expensive. The PRCs represent a source for identifying shared community and academic interests and needs. Core funding expressly earmarked for linking and enabling community-focused structures and functions would be very attractive to these institutions. The relatively low level of core funding for the PRC program and the complications of the SIP funding mechanism, however, may, in the committee's judgment, have caused some of the more research-oriented schools of public health and academic health centers to decide not to apply for funding under the PRC program. CDC could structure the program to be more attractive to institutions that have intellectual and other resources to contribute to prevention research. Further, CDC could develop a process to involve PRCs in the formulation of SIPs. If some or all of the announcements for SIPs were focused on helping PRCs to build on current work or to move research programs forward, deans and faculty members might be more motivated to establish PRCs.

SUMMARY AND CONCLUSIONS

The committee's review indicates that CDC's management of the PRC program has been creative in the face of limited resources relative to its mandate; dogged in pursuit of the mandate over a ten-year period in a bureaucratic environment that was not created or structured for the management of university-based research programs; and skilled in enhancing a sense of community and networking among the funded centers in a time of disappointing funding levels. CDC has fulfilled its initial mandate of "establishing and maintaining centers collaborating through research and demonstration to help fulfill prevention goals consistent with regional and national priorities" (PL 98-551, 1984). By further strengthening the PRC program, the CDC can increase its capacity to contribute to local, state, and national efforts to improve the health of Americans.

References

Beam D. 1982. Fragmentation of Knowledge: An Obstacle to Its Full Utilization. In KE Boulding and L Senesh, eds., *The Optimum Utilization of Knowledge: Making Knowledge Serve Human Betterment*. Boulder, Col..: Westview.

Campbell D. 1987. Guidelines for Monitoring the Scientific Competence of Preventive Intervention Research Centers: An Exercise in the Sociology of Scientific Validity. *Knowledge: Creation, Diffusion, Utilization* 8(3):389–430.

CDC (Centers for Disease Control and Prevention). n.d. *CDC Vision: Healthy People in a Healthy World Through Prevention.* Atlanta, Ga.: CDC.

CDC. 1994. *Strategic Thinking at the Centers for Disease Control and Prevention.* Atlanta, Ga.: CDC.

CDC. 1987. *Conference Summary: First National Conference on Chronic Disease Prevention and Control, Identifying Effective Strategies.* Atlanta, Ga.: CDC.

Clark NM, and McLeroy KM. 1995. Creating Capacity Through Health Education: What We Know and What We Don't. *Health Education Quarterly* 22(2):273–289.

Cousins JB, and Earl LM, eds. 1995. *Participatory Evaluation in Education: Studies in Evaluation Use and Organizational Learning.* London: Falmer.

Evans RG, and Stoddart GL. 1994. Producing Health Consuming Health Care. In RG Evans, ML Barer, and TR Marmor, eds., *Why Are Some People Healthy and Others Not? The Determinants of Health of Populations.* New York: Aldine De Gruyter, pp. 27–64.

Fals-Borda O, and Rahman MA. 1991. *Action and Knowledge: Breaking the Monopoly with Participatory Action-Research.* New York: Apex.

Fetterman DM. 1994. Empowerment Evaluation. *Evaluation Practice* 15:1–15.

Fetterman DM, Kaftarian S, and Wandersman A, eds. 1995. *Empowerment Evaluation: Knowledge and Tools for Self-Assessment and Accountability.* Beverly Hills, Calif.: Sage.

Flay BR. 1986. Efficacy and Effectiveness Trials (and Other Phases of Research) in the Development of Health Promotion Programs. *Preventive Medicine* 15:451–474.

Flay BR, and Petraitis, J. 1994. The Theory of Triadic Influence: A New Theory of Health Behavior with Implications for Preventive Interventions. In GS Albrecht, ed. *Advances in Medical Sociology, Vol IV: A Reconsideration of Models of Health Behavior Change.* Greenwich, Ct.: JAI Press, pp 19–44.

Gerstein D, and Green LW, eds. 1993. *Preventing Drug Abuse: What Do We Know?* Washington, D.C.: National Academy Press.

Green LW, George A, Daniel M, et al. 1995. *Participatory Research in Health Promotion.* Ottawa: The Royal Society of Canada.

Green LW, Kreuter MW. 1991. *Health Promotion Planning: An Educational and Environmental Approach.* Mountain View, Calif.: Mayfield.

IOM (Institute of Medicine). 1996a. *Healthy Communities: New Partnerships for the Future of Public Health.* Washington, D.C.: National Academy Press.

IOM. 1996b. *Improving Health in the Community: A Role for Performance Monitoring.* Washington, D.C.: National Academy Press.

IOM. 1988. *The Future of Public Health.* Washington, D.C.: National Academy Press.

IOM. 1984. *Responding to Health Needs and Scientific Opportunity: The Organizational Structure of the National Institutes of Health.* Washington, D.C.: National Academy Press.

Klein JT. 1985. The Evolution of a Body of Knowledge: Interdisciplinary Problem Focused Research. *Knowledge: Creation, Diffusion, Utilization* 7(2):117–142.

Koepsell TD, Wagner EH, Cheadle AC, et al. 1992. Selected Methodological Issues in Evaluating Community-Based Health Promotion and Disease Prevention Programs. *Annual Review of Public Health* 13:31–57.

Lalonde, The Honorable M. 1974. *A New Perspective on the Health of Canadians.* Ottawa, Canada: Health and Welfare.

Langton PA, ed. 1995. *The Challenge of Participatory Research: Preventing Alcohol-Related Problems in Ethnic Communities.* Washington, D.C.: Center for Substance Abuse Prevention, CSAP Cultural Competence Series 3, DHHS Pub. No. (SMA) 95-3042.

Lewin K. 1953. Studies in Group Decision. In D Cartwright, and A Zander, eds., *Group Dynamics, Research and Theory.* Evanston, Ill.: Row, Peterson.

McGinnis JM, and Foege WH. 1993. Actual Causes of Death in the U.S. *Journal of the American Medical Association* 270(18):2207–2211.

Moskowitz J, Finkelstein SN, Levy RI, et al. 1981. Biomedical Innovation: The Challenge and the Process. In J Moskowitz, SN Finkelstein, RI Levy, et al., eds., *Biomedical Innovations.* Cambridge, Ma.: MIT Press.

NAS (National Academy of Sciences), Committee on Criteria for Federal Support on Research and Development. 1995. *Allocating Federal Funds for Science and Technology.* Washington, D.C.: National Academy Press.

NCCDPHP (National Center for Chronic Disease Prevention and Health Promotion), Centers for Disease Control and Prevention, U.S. Department of Health and Human Services. 1996. *Annual Report 1996. Health Promotion and Disease Prevention Research Center Program.*

Park P, Brydon-Miller M, Hall B, et al. 1993. *Voices of Change: Participatory Research in the United States and Canada.* Toronto: Ontario Institute for Studies in Education.

Patrick DL, and Wickizer TM. 1995. Community and Health. In BC Amick, S Levine, AR Tarlov, et al., eds., *Society and Health*. New York: Oxford University Press.

Patton MQ. 1994. Developmental Evaluation. *Evaluation Practice* 15(3):311–319.

Schwartz R, and Capwell E. 1995. Advancing the Link Between Health Promotion Researchers and Practitioners: A Commentary. *Health Education Research, Theory and Practice*: i–vi.

Schwartz R, Smith C, Speers, MA, et al. 1993. Capacity Building and Resource Needs of State Health Agencies to Implement Community-Based Cardiovascular Disease Programs. *Journal of Public Health Policy* 14(4):480–494.

USDHEW (U.S. Department of Health Education and Welfare). 1979. *Healthy People*.

USDHHS (U.S. Department of Health and Human Services). 1991. *Healthy People 2000: National Health Promotion and Disease Prevention Objectives*. DHHS Pub. No. (PHS) 91-50212. Washington, D.C.: Office of the Assistant Secretary for Health.

U.S. Preventive Services Task Force, 1995.

Vertinsky I, and Vertinsky P. 1990. Resilience of Interdisciplinary Research Organizations: Case Studies of Preconditions and Life-Cycle Patterns. In PH Birnbaum-Hawe, FA Rossini, and DR Baldwin, eds., *International Research Management*. New York: Oxford University Press, pp. 31–44.

Whyte WF, ed. 1991. *Participatory Action Research*. Newbury Park, Calif.: Sage.

Appendix A

Committee Biographies

LAWRENCE W. GREEN, Dr.P.H. (*Chair*), is director of the Institute of Health Promotion Research and professor of health care and epidemiology at the University of British Columbia. Dr. Green received his degrees in public health at the University of California at Berkeley. He worked as a health educator in local, state, and federal health agencies in California and for the Ford Foundation in Dhaka, East Pakistan (now Bangladesh). During the Carter Administration, Dr. Green served as the first director of the U.S. Office of Health Information and Health Promotion. In this position, he helped coordinate the first Surgeon General's Report on Health Promotion and Disease Prevention and the 1990 Objectives for the Nation, established the National Health Information Clearinghouse, and initiated a variety of national surveys, campaigns, and federal research and demonstration programs in disease prevention and health promotion. He has served on the public health faculties at the University of California at Berkeley, The Johns Hopkins University, Harvard University, and the University of Texas. During his tenure as the Kaiser Family Foundation's vice-president and director of the health promotion program, the program received the Foundation Award of the National Association of Prevention Professionals. Dr. Green has received numerous honors and is the author of some 200 chapters, monographs, and articles. Four of his books have been widely adopted as college textbooks. He is on the editorial boards of eight journals in the health sciences, and past president of the Society for Public Health Education.

NOREEN M. CLARK, Ph.D., is dean of the University of Michigan School of Public Health and Marshall H. Becker Professor of Public Health. Her research specialty is self-management of chronic disease, and she has conducted many large-scale evaluations of health education and promotion programs. Dr. Clark has served as president of the Society for Public Health Education, and chair of the Public Health Education Section of the American Public Health Association (APHA). She is a member of the Coordinating Council of the National Asthma Education and Prevention Program. Dr. Clark is a member of the board of directors of the American Lung Association (ALA) and has chaired the ALA Technical Advisory Group on Asthma and Lung Diseases Care and Education Committee. She also serves as the editor of *Health Education Quarterly,* a preeminent scholarly journal in the field of health education. She has received the Distinguished Fellow Award, the highest honor bestowed by the Society for Public Health Education; the Derryberry Award for outstanding contribution to health education in behavioral science, given by APHA; the Health Education Research Award, conferred by the National Asthma Education Program for leadership and research contributions; and the Distinguished Career Award in Health Education and Promotion, given by APHA. Dr. Clark has extensive international experience and serves as a member of several international nonprofit organizations.

JOHN W. FARQUHAR, M.D., is director of the large, multidisciplinary Stanford Center for Research in Disease Prevention, the C. F. Rehnborg Professor of Disease Prevention in the Stanford University School of Medicine, and professor of medicine and of health research and policy. In 1971, he began the Stanford three-community study, the first controlled, comprehensive, community-based study of chronic disease prevention, followed by the ongoing Stanford five-city project. The research and dissemination methods used in these studies have been disseminated worldwide. Dr. Farquhar has received many honors including the Dana Award for Public Education, the National Cholesterol Award for Public Education, and the Research Achievement Award of the American Heart Association. Most recently he chaired the writing of the 1992 Victoria Declaration, in which international experts formulated 64 policy recommendations for worldwide reduction of cardiovascular disease. He serves as the chair of an international committee to implement the declaration's policy recommendations.

MARY DES VIGNES-KENDRICK, M.D., M.P.H., is director of the City of Houston Department of Health and Human Services. She completed her medical degree at Meharry Medical College, pediatric residency at Baylor College of Medicine, and master of public health degree at the University of Texas School of Public Health in Houston. She served as instructor and assistant professor in the department of community medicine at Baylor College of Medicine, medical director at Northside Health Center, and assistant director of personal health services at the Houston Department of Health and Human Services. Dr. des Vignes-Kendrick is board-certified in pediatrics. She is involved in public health issues at the local, state, and national levels and is the 1996 president of the National Association of County and City Health Officials.

IRA S. MOSCOVICE, Ph.D., is a professor and associate director of the Institute for Health Services Research at the University of Minnesota. He has written extensively on the use of health services research to improve health policy decisionmaking in state government and rural health care delivery systems. He is director of the Rural Health Research Centers at the University of Minnesota, funded by the Federal Office of Rural Health Policy and the Agency for Health Care Policy and Research. In 1992, he was the first recipient of the National Rural Health Association's Distinguished Researcher Award. Dr. Moscovice received his doctoral degree in operations research from Yale University.

JAMES O. PROCHASKA, Ph.D., is director of the Cancer Prevention Research Consortium and professor of clinical and health psychology at the University of Rhode Island. He is the author of over 100 publications, including three books. Dr. Prochaska is the developer of the stage model of behavior change. He has been the principal investigator on over $40 million in research grants on prevention of cancer and other chronic diseases. Dr. Prochaska serves as a consultant to the American Cancer Society, the Centers for Disease Control and Prevention, heath maintenance organizations, major corporations, and numerous universities and research centers. He has been an invited speaker at many regional, national, and international meetings and conferences.

RANDY SCHWARTZ, M.S.P.H., is director of the division of community and family health of the Maine Department of Human Services. In this capacity he is responsible for health promotion and education, maternal and child health, dental health, and public health nursing. Mr. Schwartz oversees the community health promotion/chronic disease prevention program; the diabetes control project; cardiovascular disease prevention program; cancer prevention and control, including the breast and cervical cancer prevention and control program; and tobacco prevention and control, including a contract from the National Cancer Institute to implement the ASSIST Program (American Stop Smoking Intervention Study for Cancer Prevention) in Maine, for which he is the principal investigator. Other programs for which Mr. Schwartz is responsible are teen and young adult health, injury and disabilities prevention, prenatal preventive programs, oral health, nutrition, and administrative support for public health nursing. He also served as director of the diabetes control project, which is widely recognized for its pioneering work in third-party coverage for diabetes self-management education. Mr. Schwartz has written and spoken on community interventions for health promotion, third-party reimbursement and financing for health education, quality assurance for health promotion and education, and policy and advocacy approaches in health promotion. He is past president of the Association of State and Territorial Chronic Disease Program Directors and the Association of State and Territorial Directors of Health Promotion and Public Health Education, and is the president of the Society for Public Health Education. He is also a member of the *Health*

Education Quarterly and the journal, *Family and Community Health.* He was a guest editor of the 1995 *Health Education Quarterly* theme issue on "Policy Advocacy Interventions for Health Promotion and Education." He has a master of science in public health degree from the University of Massachusetts, Amherst, and a bachelor of science degree with a concentration in community and school health education from the State University of New York at Stony Brook.

LEE SECHREST, Ph.D., is professor of psychology at the University of Arizona. He has held previous positions at Pennsylvania State University, Northwestern University, Florida State University, and the University of Michigan. He was head of the department of pychology at the University of Arizona from 1984–1989 and was director of the Center for Research on the Utilization of Scientific Knowledge at the University of Michigan from 1980–1984. He has served as president of the divisions of clinical psychology and evaluation, measurement, and statistics of the American Psychological Association and of the American Evaluation Association.

HAROLD C. SOX, JR., MD., is chairman of the department of medicine and the Joseph M. Huber Professor of Medicine at Dartmouth Medical School. He is a graduate of Stanford University and Harvard Medical School. After completing a residency at Massachusetts General Hospital, he spent two years conducting research in immunology at the National Institutes of Health and three years at Dartmouth Medical School, where he served as chief medical resident and began his studies of medical decisionmaking. Dr. Sox then spent 15 years on the faculty of Stanford University School of Medicine, where he served as chief of the division of general internal medicine and director of ambulatory care at the Palo Alto Medical Center. He returned to Dartmouth as Joseph M. Huber Professor of Medicine and chair of the department of medicine in 1988. Dr. Sox directs the Robert Wood Johnson Foundation Generalist Physician Initiative at Dartmouth. He is a regent of the American College of Physicians and chairs its education committee. Dr. Sox recently chaired the U.S. Preventive Services Task Force and the Institute of Medicine Committee to Study HIV Transmission Through Blood Products. He was elected to the Institute of Medicine of the National Academy of Sciences in 1993. His books include *Medical Decision Making* and *Common Diagnostic Tests: Selection and Interpretation.* He is a member of the editorial board of the *New England Journal of Medicine* and is an associate editor of *Scientific American Medicine.*

KENNETH E. WARNER, Ph.D., is the Richard D. Remington Collegiate Professor of Public Health in the department of health management and policy, University of Michigan School of Public Health. He is also associate director of the University's Robert Wood Johnson Foundation Clinical Scholars Program. An economist, Dr. Warner has focused his research on economic and policy aspects of disease prevention and health promotion, with a special emphasis on smoking and health. He served as the senior scientific editor of the 25th anniversary surgeon general's report on smoking and health, *Reducing the Health Consequences of Smoking: 25 Years of Progress.* Dr. Warner has been cited twice by Delta Omega, the national public health honorary society, for "outstanding achievement in public health." He received the Surgeon General's Medallion from Dr. C. Everett Koop in 1989. In 1990, he received the Leadership Award of the Alcohol, Tobacco, and Other Drugs Section of the American Public Health Association. In 1991, Dr. Warner was elected to a four-year term as a senior fellow in the Michigan Society of Fellows. He was a senior fellow at the University of Michigan's Institute of Gerontology in 1989–1990, a Kellogg national fellow from 1980 to 1983, and a visiting scholar at the National Bureau of Economic Research at Stanford University during 1975–1976. In 1996 he was elected to the Institute of Medicine and named a fellow of the Association for Health Services Research.

Appendix B

Charge to the Committee

In response to a request from CDC, the Institute of Medicine has established a committee to evaluate the Centers program to see if the program is providing the public health community with workable strategies to address major public health problems. The committee's report will discuss and make recommendations regarding (1) the overall quality of the health promotion and disease prevention research and demonstration projects being carried out at the Prevention Centers, and (2) CDC's management and oversight of the Prevention Centers.

During its deliberations, the committee will address the following questions:

(1) How innovative is the research conducted by the Prevention Centers? To what extent are university-initiated research and demonstration projects devoted to new and significant public health issues, new intervention strategies, or new methods to improve the practice of public health?

(2) What criteria do and should CDC and the universities use to select health promotion and disease prevention research and demonstration projects and to judge their results?

(3) To what extent are the findings of the research and demonstration projects and related research disseminated? What methods are used to disseminate the results of the research and demonstration projects? Are they effective?

(4) To what extent are the findings of research and demonstration projects incorporated into prevention practice, particularly by state and local health departments?

(5) What is the appropriate balance between research supported by core center funding, special interest projects, and other research funding programs; between health promotion research and disease prevention research; and between basic research in health promotion and disease prevention and development of interventions?

Appendix C

Protocol for Site Visits and
Telephone Interviews, June 1996

Innovative research. We would like to discuss the extent to which the center has conducted innovative research, by which we mean research on new issues, new or inadequately reached populations, new approaches to reaching communities/populations, and new research methods.

1. Are there specific center research or demonstration projects that demonstrate an innovative approach? In what way are these projects innovative?

2. How do the center's structure and working relationships contribute to innovation? (PROBE: interdisciplinarity and multidisciplinarity)

3. What role has CDC played in encouraging innovative research? What activities could CDC undertake to promote innovative research? (PROBE: periodic meetings of all centers, encouraging collaboration)

Criteria for selecting and judging projects. We would like to discuss the criteria you use to select research projects. In addition, we would like to discuss the ways in which CDC communicates its program criteria to the centers.

1. Please describe the center's approach to selecting its projects. We are especially interested in hearing about the criteria and process you use.
(PROBE: Does the selection process take into consideration the potential contributions of projects to scientific understanding and to public health

practice? Does the process require community input? Does this process help achieve a balance between research activities and community activities? Does this process help achieve a diversity of populations with which the center works?)

2. Has CDC clearly communicated criteria for selecting and judging projects? Please comment on the ways in which CDC communicates its program criteria to the centers.

3. In your experience, does the SIP program alter your priorities for project selection? Do SIPs reflect your mission and priorities?

Dissemination activities. We would like to know more about the center's approach to dissemination and its activities in this area. We would also like to discuss CDC's role in sharing knowledge across the centers and beyond.

1. In general, what is your approach to dissemination of research results and advances in prevention? Does the center have an overall plan? To whom do you disseminate information? Who/what are your targets?

2. How much time, effort, and resources are dedicated to dissemination? Who is responsible for dissemination?

3. Has CDC communicated explicit guidelines or expectations for dissemination to the center?

4. What efforts have been made to share knowledge between the centers and beyond? (PROBE: Is there a forum, what opportunities exist to bring together the centers through annual meetings, long-distance learning, collaboration? What works best?)

5. Are there mechanisms to link or integrate the research findings of different centers? Is knowledge being shared between the centers? Would (is) this be beneficial? Should CDC play a role in encouraging such activities? If so, how? (PROBE: Options to consider may be funding a "think tank" or integrative

center. CDC could develop principles that encourage sharing knowledge across centers and beyond, or could mandate collaboration, integration, sharing.)

6. Do the centers play a role in CDC's dissemination activities? If so, how? Does this benefit the centers? Does it help meet the centers' missions?

Prevention practice. We would like to know the degree to which your research findings have been incorporated into prevention practice.

1. Can you provide examples where practice has been changed as a result of the center's work? Are there areas where change is likely as a result of your work?

2. What is a reasonable time frame for getting demonstration sites established? What is involved in this work?

3. What barriers exist to developing and maintaining demonstration sites, both within institutions and between institutions/community? How do you address these barriers?

4. What role have health departments and community organizations played in developing demonstration projects?

5. What role has or could CDC play in facilitating the incorporation of research findings into prevention practice? (PROBE: Is CDC missing an opportunity to link science and practice?)

Balance in funding sources. We would like to discuss core funding and SIP funding.

For mature centers:

1. How has your use of core funding changed as the center has developed and matured? (PROBE: What do you use core funding for now?) What lessons have you learned regarding the use of core funding for developing and mature centers?

2. How have the types of activities changed as a center matures? How can the change in activities be reflected in funding sources? (PROBE: What are your funding priorities now that you are mature?)

For developing centers:

1. As a relatively new center, what do you view as the most important types of activities you need to undertake to be successful?

2. Do you use core funding for such activities? (PROBE: How much of the core funding is used for nonresearch purposes such as fostering community partnerships, dissemination?)

For all centers:

3. How much congruence is there between SIP research priority areas and the mission and interests of your center? In not, what does that mean for the center? Do you apply for SIPs outside of your area of interest?

4. From the perspective of a center director, what are the opportunities and limitations of SIPs?

5. How could the SIP process be improved to better foster the centers work and mission? (PROBE: More interactive process)

Notion of a Center. We would like to discuss your notion of a "research center," in terms of function, structure and utility.

Function—In your experience as a center director, what do you see as the primary functions of a "research center"?

Utility—What is the utility of a center? What is the value added? In particular, what has the center contributed that would not have been accomplished without a center? What impact has this made (process and outcome)?

Structure—How does the structure of a center influence its effectiveness?

(PROBE: Is there a typology of centers: (a) magnet for drawing in coinvestigators; (b) dispersal/dissemination entity; (c) entity for leveraging other sources of funding?)

CDC management of the program. We would like to discuss ways in which CDC can better manage the program to optimize the research conducted by centers and the impact of the centers on prevention practice.

1. In your opinion, is the relationship between universities and communities changing? If so, in what ways? Will this be important for CDC's planning for the center program during the next decade?

2. What could CDC do to better promote innovative research?

3. What could CDC do to better promote dissemination efforts?

4. What could CDC do to better facilitate the incorporation of research findings into prevention practice?

5. What could CDC do to provide funding in a way that would optimize the potential of new and mature centers to have an impact on health promotion and disease prevention?

6. Are there any other suggestions you have for ways in which CDC can strengthen the centers program? In particular, could CDC take actions to help new centers succeed and become mature centers and to assist mature centers in continuing to make contributions?

Columbia University\Harlem Hospital, June 24, 1996.

Participants included Barbara Barlow, Mary Bassett, Colin Bull, Jerry Hoke, Harold Freeman, Donald Gemson, Jean Ford, Mindy Fullilove, Robert Fullilove, Diane MacLean, Judith Butler McFie, Mary Northridge, Rev. Theodore Parker, Muriel Pettioni, Allan Rosenfield MD, Joann Toran, Goldie Watkins, Joyce Moon Howard, Steve Robinson, Harmon Moats, and Carol Roberts

University of North Carolina at Chapel Hill, June 25, 1996.

Participants included Alan Cross, Carolyn Crump, Harry Herrick, Michel Ibrahim, Miriam Settle, Michael Simmons, Ethel Jackson, and Caroline Spivey.

University of New Mexico, June 27, 1996.

Participants included Peggy Allen, Karen Arviso, Janette Carter, Leslie Cunningham-Sabo, Sally Davis, Stewart Duban, Sue Foster-Cox, Bill Freeman, Felicia Garcia, Clark Hansbarger, Deborah Helitzer-Allen, Carla Herman, Vivian Heyward, Leona Magdalena, Renate Mahler, Charlotte Morgan, Shirley Murphy, Lenora Olson, Lydia Pendley, Don Reece, Nancy Risenhoover, and Lawrence Shorty.

Prevention Research Center Directors and Co-Directors who Participated in telephone interviews.

Cheryl Alexander, Robert Anderson, Mary Bassett, William Baldyga, Ross Brownson, Alan Cross, Sally Davis, Brian Flay, Donald Gemson, Darwin Labarthe, Elisa Lee, Susan Levy, Carol Macera, Kenneth McLeroy, Joel Moskowitz, Gilbert Omenn, Guy Parcel, James Raczynski, Nancy Risenhoover, Allan Rosenfield, Miriam Settle, Kenneth Simon, Ira Tager, O. Dale Williams, and Kathleen Wright

PROTOCOL FOR SITE VISIT to CDC
June 1996

Notion of a Center. We would like to discuss your notion of a "research center," in terms of function, structure and utility.

Function—In your experience, what do you see as the primary functions of a "research center"?

Utility—What can be the utility of a center? What can be the value added? In particular, what can the centers program contributed that could not be accomplished without it? What impact has this made (process and outcome)?

Structure—How can the structure of a center influence its effectiveness?

(PROBE: Is there a typology of centers: (a) magnet for drawing in coinvestigators; (b) dispersal/dissemination entity; and (c) entity for leveraging other sources of funding?)

Innovative research. We would like to discuss the extent to which the center has conducted innovative research by which we mean research on new issues, new or inadequately reached populations, new approaches to reaching communities/populations, and new research methods.

1. Are there specific research or demonstration projects that demonstrate an innovative approach? In what way are these projects innovative?

2. What role has CDC played in encouraging innovative research? What activities could CDC undertake to promote innovative research?
(PROBE: periodic meetings of all centers, encouraging collaboration)

Criteria for selecting and judging projects. We would like to discuss the criteria you use to select and judge centers. In addition, we would like to discuss the ways in which CDC communicates its program criteria to the centers.

1. Please describe CDC's approach to selecting centers. We are especially interested in hearing about the criteria and process you use.

(PROBE: Does the selection process take into consideration the potential contributions of centers to scientific understanding and to public health practice? Does the process require community input? Does this process help achieve a balance between research activities and community activities? Does this process help achieve a diversity of populations with which the center works?)

2. Has CDC clearly communicated criteria for selecting and judging projects? Please comment on the ways in which CDC communicates its program criteria to the centers.

Dissemination activities. We would like to know more about CDC's role in sharing knowledge across the centers and beyond.

1. In general, what is your approach to dissemination of research results and advances in prevention? What role do the center play in your overall dissemination plan? To whom do you disseminate information? Who/what are your targets?

2. Has CDC communicated guidelines or expectations for dissemination to the center?

3. What efforts have been made to share knowledge between the centers and beyond? (PROBE: Is there a forum, what opportunities exist to bring together the centers through annual meetings, long distance learning, collaboration? What works best?)

4. Are there mechanisms to link or integrate the research findings of different centers? Is knowledge being shared between the centers? Would (is) this be beneficial? Should CDC play a role in encouraging such activities? If so, how? (PROBE: Options to consider may be funding a "think tank" or integrative center. CDC could develop principles that encourage sharing knowledge across centers and beyond, or could mandate collaboration, integration, sharing.)

Public health practice. We would like to know the degree to which research findings from the centers have been incorporated into public health practice.

1. Can you provide examples where public health practice has been changed as a result of the center's work? Are there areas where change is likely as a result of your work?

2. What role has or could CDC play in facilitating the incorporation of research findings into prevention practice?
(PROBE: Is CDC missing an opportunity to link science and practice?)

Balance in funding sources. We would like to discuss core funding and SIP funding

1. For new center, what do you view as the most important types of activities that should be undertaken?

2. How does the use of core funding change as the center develops and matures? (PROBE: What do you use core funding for now?) What lessons have you learned regarding the use of core funding for developing and mature centers?

3. How much congruence is there between SIP research priority areas and the missions and interests of the centers?

4. What are the opportunities and limitations of SIPs relative to other funding mechanisms?

5. How could the SIP process be improved to better foster the centers work and mission?

(PROBE: Could there be more lead time?—Perhaps a list of "tentative" project areas could be distributed early for discussion.
Could there be more "network" SIPs, which seem to work well for centers in that they allow the topic to be framed with input from centers?
Could the reviews be improved?—Centers have stated that the reviews are very general and do not provide useful feedback. At times, the quality of the review is lacking—erroneous comments supplied. Some centers think specific SIPs are "wired," leading to wasted efforts in proposal development.)

SIP Funding

1. How did you become involved in funding a SIP?

2. Please describe the topic, development of the RFA, the type of proposals you received, and the selection process. (PROBE: Was the project "wired" for a specific center? Did centers play a role in crafting the RFA?)

3. Which center was awarded the SIP? What was your experience with the project?

4. Have you been involved in other SIP projects? Would you consider working with the centers program again?

5. From the perspective, what are the opportunities and limitations of SIPs relative to other funding mechanisms?

6. How could the SIP process be improved to better serve your purpose and to foster the centers work and mission?

(PROBE: Could there be more lead time?—Perhaps a list of "tentative" project areas could be distributed early for discussion.
Could there be more "network" SIPs, which seem to work well for centers in that they allow the topic to be framed with input from centers?
Could the reviews be improved?—Centers have stated that the reviews are very general and do not provide useful feedback.
At times, the quality of the review is lacking—erroneous comments supplied. Some centers think specific SIPs are "wired" and this information is not communicated to all centers, leading to wasted efforts in proposal development.)

CDC Atlanta, July 2, 1996

Participants included the following staff from CDC: James Barrow, Don Benken, Barbara Bewerse, Sarah Kuester, Dan Miller, David McQueen, Kate McQueen, Michael Pratt, Patricia Riley, and Jean Smith.

Appendix D

The CDC Prevention Research Centers Program: A Decade of Achievement, 1986–1996, and an Agenda for the Decade Ahead

This appendix reproduces a report prepared in 1996 by the CDC Prevention Research Center directors, under the leadership of Darwin Labarthe.

THE CDC PREVENTION RESEARCH CENTERS PROGRAM:

A DECADE OF ACHIEVEMENT, 1986-1996
and
AN AGENDA FOR THE DECADE AHEAD

A landmark event for health research in the United States was the establishment of the Centers for Research and Demonstration of Health Promotion and Disease Prevention, through Public Law 98-551, enacted on October 30, 1984, and implemented by the Centers for Disease Control and Prevention (CDC) in 1986. This report illustrates the Program's achievements in its first 10 years, 1986-1996, and proposes an agenda for its further development over the next 10 years.

▲

EXECUTIVE SUMMARY

▼

The CDC Prevention Research Centers Program is unique in the nation's health research enterprise: This Program applies current knowledge about health promotion and disease prevention directly to the benefit of the public's health. And it forges essential new linkages for health between participating academic health centers and numerous federal, state, and local agencies — public and private — and with the communities they serve.

Its mission is to provide a rigorous scientific underpinning for health promotion and disease prevention policies and practices and to translate this science into the practical demonstration and evaluation of cost-effective strategies. The Program's success is a consequence of the joint efforts of CDC, state and local health departments, and their natural partners — the schools of public health and other academic health centers.

Collectively, this collaborative program of research, demonstration, and implementation of health promotion and disease prevention in local communities is having a significant impact on the nation's health.

The Critical Need for "Prevention Research"

Prevention research involves the direct and immediate application of effective strategies to benefit the public's health. Further, it aims to avert the onset of disease or disability, to reverse subclinical or inapparent disease, and to delay progression from established asymptomatic conditions to overt clinical disease and disability. The ultimate benefit of prevention research is to prolong health, well-being and self-sufficiency and thereby to enhance productivity and quality of life.

These fundamental aspects of prevention research contrast sharply with research in the laboratory and with individual patients. In fact, it is prevention research which identifies and demonstrates those products of laboratory and patient-oriented research which can be translated into direct improvements in the nation's health. Without prevention research, those other research accomplishments may remain on the shelf and thus confer no health benefit to the nation.

Achievements of the Program: 1986-1996

As of 1996 the Prevention Research Centers Program comprises 13 academic centers located as shown (see map), reflecting growth from the 3 initial Centers.[1,2] For the purposes of this report, the most significant achievements of the Program as a whole are illustrated by several brief examples:

▲ HIV/AIDS research in nine counties based at the Center for Health Promotion and Disease Prevention, University of North Carolina, Chapel Hill, has provided new information on knowledge and attitudes of religious leaders, instructional materials for care-givers, educational materials for schools, and a community resource guide, all of which serve as models for use by other agencies.

▲ Studies of disability prevention among older Americans by the Northwest Prevention Effectiveness Center, University of Washington, have demonstrated that low-cost group exercise programs in community-based senior centers can produce meaningful and measurable improvements in endurance, flexibility, lower body strength, self-reported health status, and fewer injurious falls; these findings have great potential for prolonging self-sufficiency and independent living, thereby adding to quality of life and reducing health care costs.

▲ Studies of the health of children, in order to prevent obesity, diabetes, heart attack, stroke, and other adult diseases, conducted by the Southwest Center for Prevention Research in the University of Texas-Houston Health Science Center have shown that at age 10, Mexican-American children already show a greater tendency toward risk of obesity, diabetes, heart attack, and stroke than their non-Hispanic classmates; this finding adds to information on the high risk of Mexican-

American adults and underscores the need for prevention in the school years for all children if the major burdens of adult cardiovascular diseases — personal, social and economic — are to be reduced.

▲ The special role of the Prevention Research Centers in training of public health professionals has been recognized by the Association of Schools of Public Health, which has utilized the Centers for selection and placement of its graduate public health interns; this approach capitalizes on the strengthened linkages of these Centers with the health departments where interns are placed.

▲ The Special Interest Projects (SIP) mechanism initiated by CDC matches research priorities of Centers within CDC with the capabilities of the Prevention Research Centers; multiple partnerships have now become established as a result, and for FY 1995-96 the investment of CDC in these projects reached $9.5 million; examples include the Tobacco Control Network, Support to Historically Black Colleges and Universities, and Physical Activity in Minority Women.

▲ New linkages between academic health centers and communities are illustrated by Columbia University's Harlem Center for Health Promotion and Disease Prevention, uniquely based in a community hospital (Harlem Hospital) and providing direct access to high-risk populations of New York City, in a close interaction between the University and the community developed directly through this Program.

▲ The Prevention Research Centers have multiplied the investment in research projects by being resourceful and highly effective in utilizing core funds to develop proposals for independent prevention research support; the number of prevention research projects being undertaken as a result is well above that possible with the limited core funding available to date.[3]

These achievements and many others indicate the present capacity of the Prevention Research Centers Program to fulfill its mission of research and demonstration of health promotion and disease prevention.

It is important to note that core support for this Program has remained at approximately $0.5 million per year per Center (total cost, including institutional indirect cost) since its inception. The original authorization of $1 million per Center (in 1984 dollars) has never been realized, as priority has consistently been placed on inclusion of new Centers whenever the appropriation was increased. This strategy has increased the number of Centers, which enhances the Program's impact; however, it has also limited the individual Centers' ability to conduct the full-scale demonstration and evaluation projects originally contemplated.

Meanwhile, support of background studies, pilot projects, analysis of existing data and preparation of formal research proposals has been a critical investment of the core funds awarded to each Prevention Research Center and remains a unique and indispensable feature of the Program. No alternative mechanism is available to support these preparatory research activities, which are essential for innovation in prevention research.

The Agenda for a Second Decade of Success

As of 1996, the Prevention Research Centers are demonstrably effective in generating new knowledge and applications for the benefit of the public's health. It is important to capitalize on the progress to date and to enhance the linkages that tie together CDC, state health and education agencies, and the participating academic health centers. The Program objectives presented in the table below have therefore been adopted for the decade from 1996-2006.

The Prevention Research Centers can help insure that expenditures for health care are contained wherever possible by prevention of costly illness and disability, and that expenditures for prevention are based on cost-effective evaluations of the interventions. In short, the need for prevention research is now more critical than ever before. Expanded support will allow the Prevention Research Centers to:

▲ **add continuously to knowledge of effective health promotion and disease prevention strategies for the health benefit of the public,** helping to achieve the measurable objectives of the nation's blueprint for action, **Healthy People 2000;**

▲ **expand the professional capacity to conduct prevention research and apply its results in** communities throughout the nation;

▲ **broaden and strengthen the linkages among federal, state and local health agencies and academic health centers** to improve the identification, evaluation, and application of measures for health promotion and disease prevention; and

▲ **insure that prevention research serves its critical role** complementary to laboratory and patient-oriented investigations, as part of the full spectrum of biomedical and community health research.

THE CDC PREVENTION RESEARCH CENTERS PROGRAM:

A DECADE OF ACHIEVEMENT, 1986-1996
and
AN AGENDA FOR THE DECADE AHEAD

A landmark event for health research in the United States was the establishment of the Centers for Research and Demonstration of Health Promotion and Disease Prevention, through Public Law 98-551, enacted on October 30, 1984, and implemented by the Centers for Disease Control and Prevention (CDC) in 1986. This report illustrates the Program's achievements in its first 10 years, 1986-1996, and proposes an agenda for its further development over the next 10 years.

▲

FULL REPORT
▼

Summary

▲ **The Prevention Research Centers Program is unique in the nation's health research enterprise:** Its mission is to provide a rigorous scientific underpinning for health promotion and disease prevention policies and practices and to translate this science into the practical demonstration and evaluation of cost-effective strategies.

▲ Collectively, this collaborative program of research, demonstration, and implementation of health promotion and disease prevention in local communities is having a **significant impact on the nation's health.** Examples of significant progress through this Program include studies of **HIV/AIDS, disability prevention among older Americans, and the prevention of obesity, diabetes, heart attack and stroke beginning in childhood.**

▲ Additional successes include **expanded training capacity** for public health professionals; **broadened partnerships** among components of CDC, the Prevention Research Centers, state and local health departments, and communities; and **multiplication of the investment in prevention research** by effective use of Program core funds.

▲ These achievements and many others indicate the present **capacity of the Prevention Research Centers Program to fulfill its mission** of research and demonstration of health promotion and disease prevention.

▲ Support of background studies, pilot projects, analysis of existing data, and preparation of formal research proposals has been a critical investment of the **core funds awarded to each Prevention Research Center — a unique and indispensable feature of the Program.** No alternative mechanism is available to support these preparatory research activities, which are essential for innovation in prevention research.

▲ Four Program objectives for the period 1996-2006 are proposed:

1.   Expand the level of core support per Center and the number of Centers.

2.   Broaden and strengthen the networks and interactions already developing.

3.   Establish a forum for systematic evaluation of current issues in prevention research, using Prevention Priority Panels.

4.   Reassess progress in midcourse: Reassessment, 2001 — the 15-year mark.

The collaborators in the Prevention Research Centers Program are pleased to **acknowledge the interest and participation of many individuals, organizations, agencies, and communities in the conduct of our work** and anticipate expanded cooperation toward improving the public's health in the decade ahead.

Introduction

The CDC Prevention Research Centers Program is unique in the nation's health research enterprise: This Program **applies current knowledge about health promotion and disease prevention directly to the benefit of the public's health.** And it **forges essential new linkages for health between participating academic health centers and numerous federal, state, and local agencies — public and private — and with the communities they serve.**

Its mission is to provide a rigorous scientific underpinning for health promotion and disease prevention policies and practices and to translate this science into the practical demonstration and evaluation of cost-effective strategies. The Program's success is a consequence of the joint efforts of CDC, state and local health departments, and their natural partners — the schools of public health and other academic health centers. Collectively, this collaborative program of research, demonstration, and implementation of health promotion and disease prevention in local communities is having a significant impact on the nation's health.

The Background of Program Authorization and Implementation

In July, 1981, D. A. Henderson (Dean of the Johns Hopkins School of Public Health) proposed in Congressional testimony "a national network of academic centers for health promotion and disease prevention . . . charged with education of [public health] program leaders and staff, participation in operative programs with relevant public and private agencies, and research to assess programs, to identify and measure risks and to devise new means to prevent disease."

The ensuing efforts of William F. Bridger, Robert W. Day, and Michael Gemmell, on behalf of the Association of Schools of Public Health, and the support of key members of Congress, led to the authorization of this Program in 1984 and the first appropriation for its implementation in 1986, with CDC as the implementing agency[1].

The Critical Need for "Prevention Research"

Prevention research involves the **direct and immediate application of effective strategies to benefit the public's health.** Further, it aims to **avert the onset of disease or disability, to reverse subclinical or inapparent disease, and to delay progression from established asymptomatic conditions to overt clinical disease and disability.** The ultimate benefit of prevention research is **to prolong health, well-being and self-sufficiency and thereby to enhance productivity and quality of life.**

These fundamental aspects of prevention research contrast sharply with research in the laboratory and with individual patients. In fact, it is prevention research which identifies and demonstrates those products of laboratory and patient-oriented research which can be translated into direct improvements in the nation's health. Without prevention research, those other research accomplishments may remain on the shelf and thus confer no health benefit to the nation.

The health research spectrum must extend from laboratory and patient-oriented investigation through prevention research in order to impact the health of the community — a concept not adequately conveyed by the term "biomedical research." Congress recognized the critical place of prevention research in this spectrum when it established this Program. It is timely for the health research spectrum to embrace **"biomedical and community health research."**

In addition to undertaking prevention research as described above, each Prevention Research Center is charged with bridging the health and behavioral sciences with the economic and business sectors through new *"multidisciplinary interactions"*: conducting *"developmental prevention research"* on newly-emerging issues; and providing *"shared expertise"* to health and education agencies engaged in planning and evaluation of health interventions.

With these tasks in view, CDC solicited competing applications from qualifying academic health centers throughout the United States in April, 1986.

Achievements of the Program: 1986-1996

As of 1996 the Prevention Research Centers Program comprises 13 academic centers (Table 1) located as shown (see map, Figure 1), reflecting growth from the three initial Centers. [2,3] For the purposes of this report, the most significant achievements of the Program as a whole are described, from the perspective of all 13 Centers, in five key areas:

▲ *conducting prevention research* in areas identified in the National Health Promotion and Disease Prevention Objectives;

▲ *expanding education and training resources* in prevention research;

▲ *broadening collaborations between the Prevention Research Centers and CDC;*

▲ *forging new linkages for prevention research* at local, regional and national levels[4]; and

▲ *leveraging core support to increase research capacity.*

Several brief examples illustrate these achievements:

▲ **HIV/AIDS research in nine counties** based at the Center for Health Promotion and Disease Prevention, University of North Carolina, Chapel Hill, has provided new information on knowledge and attitudes of religious leaders, instructional materials for care-givers, educational materials for schools, and a community resource guide, all of which serve as models for use by other agencies.

▲ **Studies of disability prevention among older Americans** by the Northwest Prevention Effectiveness Center, University of Washington, have demonstrated that low-cost group exercise programs in community-based senior centers can produce meaningful and measurable improvements in endurance, flexibility, lower body strength, self-reported health status, and fewer injurious falls; these findings have great potential for prolonging self-sufficiency and independent living, thereby adding to quality of life and reducing health care costs.

▲ **Studies of the health of children, in order to prevent obesity, diabetes, heart attack, stroke, and other adult diseases,** conducted by the SouthWest Center for Prevention Research in the University of Texas-Houston Health Science Center have shown that at age 10, Mexican-American children already show a greater tendency toward risk of obesity, diabetes, heart attack, and stroke than their non-Hispanic classmates; this finding adds to information on the high risk of Mexican-American adults and underscores the need for prevention in the school years for all children if the major burdens of adult cardiovascular diseases — personal, social and economic — are to be reduced.

▲ **The special role of the Prevention Research Centers in training of public health professionals** has been recognized by the Association of Schools of Public Health, which has utilized the Centers for selection and placement of its graduate public health interns;

this approach capitalizes on the strengthened linkages of these Centers with the health departments where interns are placed.

▲ **The Special Interest Projects (SIP) mechanism initiated by CDC** matches research priorities of Centers within CDC with the capabilities of the Prevention Research Centers; multiple partnerships have now become established as a result, and for FY 1995-96 the investment of CDC in these projects reached $9.5 million; examples include the Tobacco Control Network, Support to Historically Black Colleges and Universities, and Physical Activity in Minority Women (see, for example, Figure 2).

▲ **New linkages between academic health centers and communities** are illustrated by Columbia University's Harlem Center for Health Promotion and Disease Prevention, uniquely based in a community hospital (Harlem Hospital) and providing direct access to high-risk populations of New York City, in a close interaction between the University and the community developed directly through this Program.

▲ **The Prevention Research Centers have multiplied the investment in research projects** by being resourceful and highly effective in utilizing core funds to develop proposals for independent prevention research support; the number of prevention research projects being undertaken as a result is well above that possible with the limited core funding available to date.[5]

These achievements and many others indicate the present capacity of the Prevention Research Centers Program to fulfill its mission of research and demonstration of health promotion and disease prevention.

It is important to note that core support for this Program has remained at approximately $0.5 million per year per Center (total cost, including institutional indirect cost) since its inception (see Figure 2, "core"). The original authorization of $1 million per Center (in 1984 dollars) has never been realized, as priority has consistently been placed on inclusion of new Centers whenever the appropriation was increased. This strategy has increased the number of Centers, which enhances the Program's impact; however, it has also limited the individual Centers' ability to conduct the full-scale demonstration and evaluation projects originally contemplated. This level of research project — such as comprehensive community-based evaluations of the effectiveness and cost-benefit of new interventions — must await increased funding in the future.

Meanwhile, support of background studies, pilot projects, analysis of existing data, and preparation of formal research proposals has been a critical investment of the core funds awarded to each Prevention Research Center and remains a unique and indispensable feature of the Program. No alternative mechanism is available to support these preparatory research activities, which are essential for innovation in prevention research.

To assure the continued success of the Program, core funding must be continued and, insofar as possible, increased to strengthen the existing Centers and to maintain the momentum of growth experienced in the first 10 years.

The Agenda for a Second Decade of Success

As of 1996, the Prevention Research Centers are demonstrably effective in generating new knowledge and applications for the benefit of the public's health. It is important to capitalize on the progress to date and to enhance the linkages that tie together CDC, state health and education agencies, and the participating academic health centers.

The Prevention Research Centers can help insure that expenditures for health care are contained wherever possible by prevention of costly illness and disability, and that expenditures for prevention are based on cost-effective evaluations of the interventions. In short, the need for prevention research is now more critical than ever before. Expanded support will allow the Prevention Research Centers to:

▲ *add continuously to knowledge of effective health promotion and disease prevention strategies for the health benefit of the public,* helping to achieve the measurable objectives of the Public Health Service blueprint, Healthy People 2000;

▲ *expand the professional capacity to conduct prevention research and apply its results in* communities throughout the nation;

▲ *broaden and strengthen the linkages among federal, state and local health agencies and academic health centers* needed to improve the identification, evaluation, and application of measures for health promotion and disease prevention; and

▲ *insure that prevention research serves its critical role* complementary to laboratory and patient-oriented investigations, as part of the full spectrum of biomedical and community health research.

Program Objectives, 1996-2006

The agenda for the second decade of the CDC Prevention Research Centers Program includes four specific objectives (each objective is addressed briefly below):

1. ***Expand the level of core support per Center and the number of Centers.***

2. ***Broaden and strengthen the networks and interactions* which are already developing.**

3. ***Establish a forum for systematic evaluation of current issues* in prevention research, using Prevention Priority Panels.**

4. ***Reassess progress in midcourse:* Reassessment, 2001 – the 15-year mark.**

1. Expand the level of core support per Center and the number of Centers.

Increasing the level of core support per Center to at least the level of $1 million authorized in 1984 will greatly enhance the contributions of the Program:

▲ The research, demonstration and evaluation projects on the scale contemplated in the original legislation will become feasible;

▲ training opportunities for health professional can be diversified and expanded; and

▲ the impact of the CDC, state and local health departments, and their academic and medical care partners toward achievement of the Healthy People 2000 goals and objectives will be accelerated.

Increasing the number of Centers to include at least 20 states will broaden involvement of schools of public health and other qualified academic health centers and their community-based constituencies.

2. Broaden and strengthen the networks and interactions which are already developing.

The Prevention Centers Program should continue to lead CDC beyond its traditional focus on state health departments and to bring academic health centers outside their institutional bounds to interact jointly with communities, at work sites, and in other settings. Continuation of these developments will help to:

▲ link all components of CDC with their academic partners through the Prevention Research Centers Program;

▲ build partnerships with a wider array of health, education, housing, and managed care organizations in communities throughout the country; and

▲ provide leadership for the professional organizations in medicine and public health to enhance healthful behavior and empower all Americans to take charge of their personal health and their communities' health.

3. Establish a forum for systematic evaluation of current issues in prevention research, using Prevention Priority Panels.

Prevention Priority Panels should be appointed by CDC and the network of Prevention Research Centers on a biennial basis to review science and policy on specific questions of national importance in health promotion and disease prevention, including gaps in current policies, needs for legislative initiatives, or priorities for further research.

4. Reassess progress in midcourse: Reassessment, 2001, the 15-year mark.

The next formal internal Program reassessment should address progress toward achievement of the foregoing Program objectives, using the following criteria for success:

▲ the impacts of the Prevention Research Centers on community health measures, as presented in *Healthy People 2000;*

▲ the adequacy of the number of Centers and their level of core support;

▲ the strength and breadth of Program linkages with multiple component s of CDC and with professional organizations dedicated to prevention;

▲ the contribution of the initial Prevention Priority Panels to resolution of issues in prevention research and prevention practice; and

▲ the quality of the Program's contributions in the areas of new knowledge, new applications, new training programs and opportunities, and new partnerships for effective health promotion and disease prevention.

Acknowledgments

The collaborators in the Prevention Research Centers Program are pleased to acknowledge the interest and participation of many individuals, organizations, agencies, and communities in the conduct of our work and anticipate expanded cooperation toward improving the public's health in the decade ahead.

The Prevention Research Center Directors, in presenting this report, wish especially to acknowledge those whose efforts brought about the establishment of this program:

First, Dr. D.A. Henderson, formerly Dean of the Johns Hopkins University School of Public Health, for proposing the concept before a hearing chaired by Sen. Orrin Hatch in 1981 and Dr. Robert Day, then President of the Association of Schools of Public Health; next, Dr. William F. Bridgers, formerly Dean of the University of Alabama at Birmingham School of Public Health, for devoting countless hours on Capitol Hill in pursuit of a vision that eventually became the Prevention Centers Program — the Centers would have remained no more than proposal if not for Dr. Bridgers' relentless determination, intellectual vigor and just plain hard work; and not least, our friends and supporters on Capitol Hill — Senator Hatch and his principal health advisor, Dr. David Sundwall; Senator Kennedy and his staffer, JoAnne Glisson, to whom we owe special thanks for her keen advice and counsel; then Representative and now Senator Shelby; Representative Waxman and his staffers Dr. Brian Biles and Ruth Katz, who counseled ASPH throughout the campaign and first identified its early champions (then Representative and now Senator Mikulski and Representative Scheur); Tony McCann, then Senate Budget Committee staffer, for his assistance and counsel; and Dr. William Roper, then Special Advisor for Health to President Reagan, who signed S.771 into law, thanks to him.

Footnotes

[1] See Appendix 1: Public Law 98-551 — Oct. 30, 1984.

[2] In a detailed appendix to this report, the 13 currently funded Prevention Research Centers are characterized individually. This information includes for each Center its institutional base; its research theme; its collaborative arrangements and organizational interactions established to date; and a profile of its current prevention research projects.

[3] Three other Centers were discontinued on the basis of extensive scientific peer review.

[4] See, for example, Table 2.

[5] See National Center for Chronic Disease Prevention and Health Promotion. *Prevention Centers: Making Prevention a Practical Reality. Annual Report 1996.* U.S. Department of Health and Human Services, Public Health Service, Centers for Disease Control and Prevention. January, 1996.

FACT SHEET

THE CDC PREVENTION RESEARCH CENTERS PROGRAM:

A DECADE OF ACHIEVEMENT, 1986-1996
and
AN AGENDA FOR THE DECADE AHEAD

In a landmark event for health research in the United States, the **Prevention Research Centers Program**[1] was established through PL 98-551 (October 30, 1984).

This Program was implemented by the **Centers for Disease Control and Prevention (CDC)** in 1986. A new report illustrates the Program's achievements in its first 10 years, 1986-1996, and proposes an agenda for its further development over the next 10 years, 1996-2006.

The **Prevention Research Centers Program is unique in the nation's health research enterprise:** It applies current knowledge about health promotion and disease prevention directly to the benefit of the public's health, and it forges essential new linkages for health between participating academic health centers and numerous federal, state, and local agencies — public and private — and with the communities they serve.

The **Program mission** is to provide a rigorous scientific underpinning for health promotion and disease prevention policies and practices and to translate this science into the practical demonstration and evaluation of cost-effective strategies.

The **ultimate benefit of prevention research** is to test the application of promising products of laboratory and patient-oriented research in communities to determine their real impact on the public's health.

Collectively, this collaborative program of research, demonstration, and implementation of health promotion and disease prevention in local communities is having a **significant impact on the nation's health.** Examples of significant progress through this Program include studies of **HIV/AIDS, disability prevention among older Americans,** and the **prevention of obesity, diabetes, heart attack and stroke beginning in childhood.**

Additional successes include **expanded training capacity** for public health professionals; **broadened partnerships** among components of CDC, the Prevention Research Centers, state and local health departments, and communities; and **multiplication of the investment in prevention research** by effective use of core funds awarded through the Program.

These achievements and many others indicate the present **capacity of the Prevention Research Centers Program to fulfill its mission** of research and demonstration of health promotion and disease prevention.

Support of background studies, pilot projects, analysis of existing data, and preparation of formal research proposals has been a critical investment of the **core funds awarded to each Prevention Research Center — a unique and indispensable feature of the Program. No alternative mechanism is available to support these preparatory research activities, which are essential for innovation in prevention research.**

continued

PROGRAM OBJECTIVES: 1996-2006

1. Expand the level of core support per Center and the number of Centers.

Increasing the level of core support per Center to at least the level of $1 million authorized in 1984 will greatly enhance the contributions of the Program. Increasing the number of Centers to include at least 20 states will broaden involvement of schools of public health and other qualified academic health centers and their community-based constituencies.

2. Broaden and strengthen the networks and interactions which are already developing.

The Prevention Centers Program should continue to lead CDC beyond its traditional focus on state health departments and to bring academic health centers outside their institutional bounds to interact jointly with communities, at work sites, and in other settings.

3. Establish a forum for systematic evaluation of current issues in prevention research, using Prevention Priority Panels.

Prevention Priority Panels should be appointed by CDC and the network of Prevention Research Centers on a biennial basis to review science and policy on specific questions of national importance in health promotion and disease prevention, including gaps in current policies, needs for legislative initiatives, or priorities for further research.

4. Reassess progress in midcourse: Reassessment 2001, the 15-year mark.

The next formal internal Program reassessment should address progress toward achievement of the foregoing Program objectives.

---

[1]Formally, the Centers for Research and Demonstration of Health Promotion and Disease Prevention

Appendix E

Prevention Research Centers: Investing in the Nation's Health, 1986–1996

Program information prepared in 1996 by the Prevention Research Center staff at the CDC.

Prevention Research Centers:

Investing in the Nation's Health

1986–1996

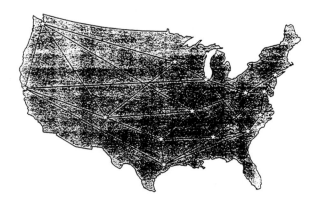

"The future health of the nation will be determined by how effectively we are able to link federal, academic, state, and local health agencies in a range of collaborative and innovative programs, like CDC's Prevention Research Centers Program, which strengthens the fabric of public health."

D. A. Henderson, M.D., M.P.H.
University Distinguished Professor and former Dean
The Johns Hopkins School of Hygiene and Public Health

 U.S. DEPARTMENT OF HEALTH AND HUMAN SERVICES
Public Health Service
Centers for Disease Control and Prevention

National Research Network

The CDC-administered Health Promotion Disease Prevention Research Centers Program integrates the resources of 14 academic centers committed to research that benefits public health. This national network for applied research focuses on the behaviors that put Americans at risk for chronic health conditions that claim a disproportionate number of lives. The centers are particularly concerned about the quality of life for special populations (including the elderly and the underserved) and how to curb the premature morbidity and mortality that drive the nation's excessive health care costs.

The expertise of university research centers is made available to health agencies, community-based organizations, and national nonprofit organizations. This link between university research and grassroots organizations helps turn research results into practical, cost-effective, and innovative programs.

> *Physical inactivity is a modifiable risk behavior linked to several chronic diseases. Not all assessments of physical activity among minority women have been appropriate for the specific population studied. The prevention centers at the University of South Carolina and the University of New Mexico are entering the second year of community-based research on physical activity practices among black and American Indian women aged 40 years or older. This effort is providing innovative survey instruments for asking respondents about the types of activities in which they are most likely to be involved—that is, activities integral to the daily lives of these women.*

High-Priority Research Themes

In 1986, the first three centers were funded, and new centers have been continually added. Research themes have broadened to include specific conditions (such as cardiovascular disease) and the health status of children and adolescents. The network now links a set of well-respected research institutes focusing on the health conditions of diverse communities in distinct geographic areas, including Harlem, the Southwest, Appalachia, and Missouri's Bootheel.

Host University	First Funded	Research Theme
University of Alabama at Birmingham	1993	▸ Risk Reduction Among African-American and Other Underserved Populations
University of California at Berkeley	1993	▸ Families, Neighborhoods, and Communities: A Model for Action in Chronic Disease Prevention
Columbia University	1990	▸ Reduction of Excess Morbidity and Mortality in the Harlem Community
University of Illinois at Chicago	1990	▸ Health Promotion and Disease Prevention Across the Lifespan
The Johns Hopkins University	1993	▸ Promoting Health and Preventing Disease Among Urban and Rural Adolescents
University of Minnesota	1996	▸ Teen Pregnancy Prevention
University of New Mexico	1995	▸ Promoting Healthy Lifestyles in American Indians
University of North Carolina at Chapel Hill	1986	▸ Workplace Health Promotion
University of Oklahoma	1994	▸ Promoting Healthy Behavior and Disease Prevention in Native American Populations
Saint Louis University	1994	▸ Cardiovascular Disease Prevention in Low-Income Rural Communities
University of South Carolina	1993	▸ Promoting Health Through Physical Activity
University of Texas at Houston	1986	▸ From Healthy Children to Healthy Adults
University of Washington at Seattle	1986	▸ Keeping Older Adults Healthy and Independent
West Virginia University	1994	▸ Risk Factors in Appalachia

Support for National Health Objectives

The prevention centers' research environment furthers four main goals that support progress in achieving national health objectives.

Maximize Resources for Complex Public Health Research

The program not only encourages extramural research in public health but creates an environment in which academic centers can communicate about and collaborate on research themes. The centers share ideas, discuss strategies, and pool talent and material resources to avoid unnecessary duplication of effort.

Each center also fosters interaction among faculty in different disciplines. Departments of education, psychology, social work, and nursing are involved with the school of public health or the preventive medicine program that oversees the prevention center. Since most health issues are complex, this blending of expertise is advantageous to finding workable solutions.

> *The Tobacco Control Network stimulates interaction among multidisciplinary staff at nearly every prevention center. The network, coordinated by the University of Illinois, collaborates with CDC's Office on Smoking and Health in selecting tobacco control research themes for the prevention centers. For example, the centers are seeking to increase understanding about adolescent smoking and the racial and geographic differences in teen smoking behavior. Researchers from behavioral science, nursing, anthropology, social work, and epidemiology are working together to find strategies that discourage tobacco use among youth. Without the structure of the prevention centers program, this multifaceted and interinstitutional interaction might not occur, and the research would be less rich.*

Make Communities Accessible and Amenable to Prevention Interventions

Long-standing relationships between the prevention centers and their immediate communities bring public health researchers closer to the public. Interventions can be introduced so that they are most effective and credible to specific populations. Multiple health risk factors can be simultaneously addressed by strategies that anticipate underlying community attitudes, beliefs, and perceptions.

> *Researchers at the University of North Carolina are surveying the health attitudes and beliefs of the black community in Durham, North Carolina. Investigators are assessing the degree to which the community trusts government-sponsored biomedical research—a preliminary evaluation that could not be done by the government itself. Results from this representative community will guide federal agencies in promoting AIDS vaccine trials and other therapies in black communities throughout the United States.*

Increase Collaboration Among Agencies and Nontraditional Partners

The program allows collaboration among federal and nonfederal partners. For example, the prevention centers program is conducting the community prevention component of the National Institutes of Health's multiyear Women's Health Initiative, one of the largest U.S. prevention studies of perimenopausal and postmenopausal women.

In addition, each prevention center must conduct at least one demonstration project with a state or local health department, board of education, or community-based organization. The University of California at Berkeley, for example, has forged partnerships with managed care alliances and health maintenance organizations (HMOs). Public health departments are using information about preventive health services among private patients to design a family HMO for economically disadvantaged families.

"The leadership from The Johns Hopkins Center for Adolescent Health Promotion and Disease Prevention has been the catalyst for bringing together local organizations serving youth. The center's one-day conference, 'Best Practices in Adolescent Health,' addressed the three issues that most threaten our young people: violence, substance abuse, and injuries. Community providers shared information about their successes. This type of networking strengthens grassroots prevention programs."

Judith Sensenbrenner, M.D., M.P.H.
Health Officer, Wicomico County, Maryland

Train Public Health Professionals

By involving academic researchers; federal, state, and local public health workers; personnel from numerous national agencies and community-based organizations; and practitioners from hospitals and managed care environments, the prevention centers program is expanding the capacity of diverse professionals to conduct prevention research and apply its results. In addition, the Association of Schools of Public Health places graduate public health interns in the prevention centers. Thus, the centers are a continuous source of education and training for both current and future disease prevention researchers. The interns benefit from exposure to research that involves faculty from several academic departments and that tests innovative ways to approach public health issues.

At the University of Washington's Northwest Center for Prevention Research, the School of Public Health and Community Medicine, the School of Pharmacy, and the area's largest health maintenance organization are collaborating on a database project linking patients' pharmacologic records with patients' health status information and socio-demographic characteristics. These comprehensive patient profiles will offer researchers a unique body of data in which to test epidemiologic hypotheses. Students involved in this project are in the vanguard of the emerging partnership between the public health sector and managed care.

---

*Collaborative research concerning American Indians in one state created an extensive research network. Similar partnerships have developed around every prevention center. ***

University
| Prevention Research Center |

State Level
| Department of Health |

Community Level
| Tribal Health Board |
| Ambulatory Care Clinics in 4 Cities |
| Community Hospital |

Federal Level
| Indian Health Service |

National Nonprofit Agencies
| Heart Association |
| Diabetes Association |

* Example derived from the University of Oklahoma Center for Prevention Research in Native Americans.

4

Value-Added Funding of Prevention Research

Recognition that an investment in prevention can improve the quality of life and lead to savings in health care and other societal costs prompted the establishment of the prevention centers program by public law in 1984.

The core program dollars CDC provides constitute a small but critical percentage of each prevention center's overall budget. These dollars support each center's basic infrastructure—core faculty and research assistants—without which the center would not exist. Every prevention center has been able to leverage CDC dollars to garner additional outside support for health promotion research, demonstration projects, and the dissemination of findings. Thus, the prevention research capacity has expanded well beyond the basic level of program support.

For example, the University of Alabama's Center for Health Promotion increased its applied research capacity ninefold in three years. The additional prevention research resources were not forthcoming until CDC's initial investment had been made. Similarly, CDC's seed money for the University of Washington's Center for Health Promotion in Older Adults funded a study that in turn attracted an additional half-million dollars. At Columbia University, CDC core dollars funded only 3 of 15 prevention projects this year, and at the University of Texas, 4 of 29.

CDC's continued investment in the prevention centers sustains their core resources and their ability to attract support for wide-ranging prevention research. Interest has come from other agencies, foundations, and programs that want to invest in CDC-supported research institutes.

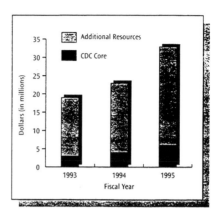

Benefits of Continuity

Sustained support ensures that research in progress remains uninterrupted and that the well-developed research network remains intact. Prevention projects can then be replicated and disseminated, prevention training for health professionals can be enhanced and diversified, and progress toward achieving national health objectives can be accelerated. Goals for the next decade of progress are designed to expand the breadth and depth of the total prevention effort.

"The arrangement affords an ideal combination of talents—a public health agency's experience in working with high-risk populations and the research skills of a health sciences center."

Bert Malone, M.P.A.
Director, Division of Chronic Disease Prevention and Health Promotion
Missouri Department of Health

"*The University of New Mexico Center for Health Promotion has helped us, as a community, maintain focus on prevention issues and total health. The direction the center provides benefits our community through our Tribal Health Department.*"

Randolph Padilla
Governor, Pueblo of Jemez, New Mexico

Extending the Public Health Mission

The prevention centers' two main program goals support and enhance CDC's public health mission.

Prevention centers' goals

▸ Provide a sound scientific basis for health promotion and disease prevention policies and practices.

▸ Translate research findings into community-based interventions.

CDC's mission

Promote health and improve the quality of life for Americans by preventing and controlling disease, injury, and disability.

Key Accomplishments

Members of the prevention centers accomplish many prevention research goals.

▸ Collaborate with academic institutions and state and local government agencies to address high-priority public health issues.

▸ Reach diverse ethnic and racial communities for collecting data and transferring results.

▸ Conduct demonstration and evaluation projects.

▸ Disseminate the latest research results.

▸ Serve as an extension of the public health effort.

▸ Expand the training capacity for public health professionals.

▸ Multiply the investment in prevention research by effectively using core funds to attract funding from other sources.

▸ Conduct background studies and pilot projects, analyze survey data, and conduct innovative prevention research.

In Missouri's Bootheel, the Saint Louis University Prevention Center translates science into practice by forging coalitions that take chronic disease prevention interventions to communities. These coalitions represent a 13-county area that is medically underserved and economically disadvantaged and has the highest rates of chronic disease in the state. The center designs interventions to address the three main risk factors among people in the area: poor diet, smoking, and physical inactivity. Working through the coalitions, the center teaches school-age youth how to eat healthily, helps local officials curb tobacco sales to minors, and builds walking trails in areas where sidewalks are infeasible. These efforts are predicated on the belief that deeply ingrained habits, traditions, and cultural norms influence disease rates and that change can be achieved only by the people themselves.

For more information, please contact:
Centers for Disease Control and Prevention
Health Promotion Disease Prevention Research
* Centers Program, Mail Stop K–30*
4770 Buford Highway, NE
Atlanta, GA 30341-3724
Phone: (770) 488-5395
E-mail: njs0@ccdosa1.em.cdc.gov

6 ▸